Making the Most of Medical School

The Alternative Guide
First Edition

Edited by
Ashton Barnett-Vanes

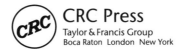

CRC Press
Taylor & Francis Group
Boca Raton London New York

CRC Press is an imprint of the
Taylor & Francis Group, an **informa** business

CRC Press
Taylor & Francis Group
6000 Broken Sound Parkway NW, Suite 300
Boca Raton, FL 33487-2742

© 2018 by Taylor & Francis Group, LLC
CRC Press is an imprint of Taylor & Francis Group, an Informa business

No claim to original U.S. Government works

Printed in Great Britain by Ashford Colour Press Ltd

International Standard Book Number-13: 978-1-138-19655-1 (Paperback)

Visit the Taylor & Francis Web site at
http://www.taylorandfrancis.com

and the CRC Press Web site at
http://www.crcpress.com

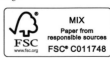

Contents

Preface

Collected on these pages is a wealth of insights, experiences and advice distilled to provide you, the reader, with a richly informative but hopefully not overwhelming series of chapters on what you can do to make the most of medical school. Too often I have witnessed students' noble ambitions – be it in research, leadership or elsewhere – squandered by a lack of experience, insight or guidance. This represents a *lose–lose* situation: students are deprived of an opportunity to build their skills or track record, often to the detriment of their future enthusiasm and engagement, and medicine or society at large is deprived of the weird and perhaps wonderful contribution they might have otherwise (one day) made. While completing medical school and becoming a safe and competent doctor is the number one goal – I hope this book will aid readers to make the most of this time and, with any luck, their careers thereafter.

Ashton Barnett-Vanes

Acknowledgements

I thank the many contributors who offered their time and experience to make this book a reality, including those who provided helpful review of other chapters: Dr Joanna Koster, my commissioning editor at Taylor & Francis, for her support from the beginning of this book, and Julia Molloy, Adel Rosario and Kyle Meyer for their tireless coordination and administration. I acknowledge Kate Pool and her team at the Society of Authors for their advice and guidance. My thanks go to students and colleagues who wittingly or otherwise gave me inspiration for this project and the many teachers and leaders who have lent their support over the years. Finally, I owe a debt of gratitude to friends and family, whose unwavering patience and generosity allowed me to take this book to completion. This book is dedicated to the memory of Jolyon Jones.

Ashton Barnett-Vanes

Editor

Dr Ashton Barnett-Vanes is a Final Year Medical Student based in London, United Kingdom. He completed his medical and clinical science years at St George's, University of London where he was awarded the William Brown and Devitt-Pendlebury Exhibition. In 2012, he graduated with first class honours in his intercalated BSc and in 2015 completed his PhD in war injuries – both at Imperial College London. He is a former intern of the World Health Organization and in 2016 was a British Council scholar at Tsinghua University, Beijing. He is the recipient of a Foulkes Foundation Fellowship.

OTHER BOOK BY THE EDITOR

How to Complete a PhD in the Medical and Clinical Sciences, Wiley–Blackwell, Hoboken, NJ, 2017.

Contributors

Osaid H. Alser MD
Junior Doctor
Islamic University of Gaza Medical School, Gaza, Palestine

Sir Sabaratnam Arulkumaran MD PhD FRCS FRCOG
Professor Emeritus of Obstetrics and Gynaecology
St George's University of London, London, UK

Jeroen van Baar BSc MSc
4th Year PhD Student
Donders Institute, Radboud University, Nijmegen, the Netherlands

Neomi Bennett BSc RGN
Nurse
Kingston University of London, Kingston, UK;
Founder
Neo-Slip, London, UK

Chris Bodimeade BA MSc
2nd Year Medical Student
University of Leicester, Leicester, UK

Ruben V. C. Buijs MD
2nd Year Resident
University of Utrecht, Utrecht, the Netherlands

Frank Chinegwundoh MBE MBBS MS MML FRCS(Eng) FRCS(Ed) FRCS(Urol) FEBU
Consultant Urological Surgeon
Barts Health NHS Trust, London, UK;
Honorary Visiting Professor
School of Health Sciences City, University of London, London, UK

Katie Dallison BSc MA
Medical Careers Consultant
British Medical Association, London, UK;
Imperial College London, London, UK

Henry D. I. De'Ath MBBS MRCS PhD
Registrar in General Surgery and Trauma
Queen Mary University of London, London, UK;
Wessex Deanery, Winchester, UK

Daniel Di Francesco MA DPMSA
4th Year Medical Student
King's College London, London, UK

Randa ElMallah MD MBBS
Resident in Orthopaedic Surgery
University of Mississippi Medical Center, Jackson, Mississippi

James Frater
2nd Year Medical Student
King's College London, London, UK

Shiv Gaglani MBA
Medical Student
Johns Hopkins School of Medicine, Baltimore, Maryland;
Co-Founder and CEO of Osmosis (https://www.osmosis.org/)

Sophia Haywood
4th Year Medical Student
University of East Anglia, Norwich, UK

Moa Herrgård
3rd Year Medical Student
Karolinska Institute, Stockholm, Sweden;
2nd Year Law Student
Stockholm University, Stockholm, Sweden

Jenny Higham MBBS MD FRCOG FHEA
Principal and Professor
St George's University of London, London, UK

Babak Javid MB BChir PhD MRCP
Professor and Principal Investigator
Tsinghua University School of Medicine, Beijing, China

Ira Kleine MA MBBS
Foundation Doctor
Royal Free London NHS Foundation Trust, London, UK

Saori Koshino MD
FY2 Doctor
University of Tokyo, Tokyo, Japan

Jonathan C. H. Lau BSc MSc
4th Year PhD Student
University of Cambridge, Cambridge, UK;
University College London, London, UK

Vernon Lee MBBS PhD MPH MBA
Associate Professor of Public Health
National University of Singapore, Singapore

Jasmin Lovestone BA
5th Year Medical Student
University of East Anglia, Norwich, UK

Azeem Majeed MD FRCP FRCGP FFPH
Professor of Primary Care
Imperial College London, London, UK

Maniragav Manimaran BSc
4th Year Medical Student
University College London, London, UK

Chris McMurran BA
MB-PhD Student
Trinity College, University of Cambridge, Cambridge, UK

Edgar Meyer BSc PhD
Associate Dean of Undergraduate Programmes
Imperial College Business School, London, UK

Andrew Papanikitas BSc MA MBBS PhD
Academic Clinical Lecturer in General Practice
University of Oxford, Oxford, UK

Rose Penfold BA BM BCh
Academic Foundation Doctor
University of Oxford, Oxford, UK;
Imperial College Healthcare NHS Trust, London, UK

Kyle Ragins MD MBA
Resident Physician
Department of Emergency Medicine
David Geffen School of Medicine at University of California,
Los Angeles

Tim Robinson BMedSci MBChB
Junior Doctor
University of Birmingham, Birmingham, UK

Jim Ryan OBE OSTJ MB MCh FRCS FRCEM
Professor Emeritus
St George's University of London, London, UK;
International Professor of Surgery
Uniformed Services University of the Health Sciences, Bethesda, Maryland

Jason Sarfo-Annin MA BM BCh MPH MRCP
Academic Clinical Fellow in Primary Care
University of Bristol, Bristol, UK

Adam Staten MA MBBS MRCP MRCGP DRCOG DMCC
General Practitioner
The Red House Surgery, Bletchley, UK

William Tamale MBChB MPH
Clinic Manager
Joint Clinical Research Centre, Lubowa, Uganda

Ada E. D. Teo BA MA PhD
MB-PhD Student
University of Cambridge, Cambridge, UK

In-Ae Tribe BSc MBBS
Clinical Teaching Fellow
Chelsea and Westminster NHS Trust, London, UK

Jonathan C. M. Wan BSc AKC
MB-PhD Student
University of Cambridge, Cambridge, UK

Wong Yisheng MBBS
Resident in Dermatology
National Skin Centre, Singapore

CHAPTER 1

Introduction

Ashton Barnett-Vanes

Without doubt, a 4- to 6-year period of study in medical school is challenging, burdensome and costly. Your *raison d'etre* during this time is the learning, understanding and application of clinical medicine – for which there are countless books already. Yet medical school can serve as a platform for more than the achievement of this, albeit essential, goal. This book is intended to serve as an alternative guide for medical students seeking to develop a wider set of skills, qualifications or experience in areas relevant to today's and tomorrow's clinical world. While it is intended to be read primarily by medical students, it is likely that junior doctors and other healthcare professionals in training or early practice will find this book of use.

Today, training programmes in medicine and surgery are placing increasing expectations on the non-clinical attributes medical students and junior doctors must possess and demonstrate for job competitiveness. They include – inter alia – academic publications and presentations, leadership skills, teaching experience, policy and management training – to name just a few. Medical students and those in the early stages of training can feel under pressure to acquire as many of these attributes as possible. But like most things in life that are worthwhile, rushing is ill advised. Accordingly, this book seeks to go beyond the tick box-style nature of today's 'curriculum vitae (CV) building', to offer thoughtful guidance and advice from writers with real-life experience as, or teaching, students.

For instance, scrambling around a poorly conceived research idea is unlikely to even bring good data, never mind an academic publication. If your eyes are fixated on the output, you risk overlooking arguably the most important part of the endeavour at this stage: understanding the *process*. Becoming a successful researcher does not depend on how many papers or letters you have on PubMed, but whether you can see problems, hypothesise a cause and construct a methodical approach to solving them – or at least proving they exist, as covered in Chapter 2.

Alongside research and academic skills, medical school offers a unique opportunity to both observe and demonstrate leadership and organisational acumen. In Chapter 3, two common examples are outlined – establishing a group or campaign and organising an event, told through the experience of running a conference. These chapters cover a wealth of insight and lessons learned but, importantly, impart advice that the reader can mould and apply to a diverse range of activities outside of the remit of this book – a feature central to its wider function. Communication is central to the advancement of medicine, and Chapter 4 focusses on core topics in this area such as writing and publishing books, blogging and authoring for the general public and public speaking and presentations – the latter covering a range of scenarios that are featured in chapters elsewhere.

Chapter 5 focusses on the opportunities medical school offers for international health exchange and learning told through medical electives, global health research and internships. Importantly, this chapter includes a diverse collection of perspectives and insights from both high- and low-resource settings. Although the elective sections are written with the view of going abroad, much of their contents are readily transferrable to a domestic adventure. Chapter 6 explores the breadth of further degrees one can consider during and after medical school, and while not exhaustive, it is certainly comprehensive. Elsewhere, chapters cover opportunities in medical education, law and ethics and innovation and management. Chapter 9 covers an area of increasing interest – international mobility in medical training and practice. Finally, Chapter 10 features career perspectives from eminent clinicians who have combined the demands of clinical practice with exemplary leadership in their field.

In closing, this book is to be used and not just read. Annotate it, make notes, even cross out things you do not agree with: if it is not falling apart at the seam by the time you are finished with it, something is not right. Finally, while it is important to develop and lead a rich and fulfilling life as a student and beyond, keep your eyes on the prize. The completion of medical school and your graduating as a doctor is the number one aim. Striking a balance between curricular and extracurricular activities is vital – don't overdo it!

So without further ado, welcome to the first *Alternative Guide to Medical School*.

Box 1.1   Undergraduate's perspective

Being exposed to the health challenges in Jamaica was a catalyst in deciding to find a career where I could help people. This, coupled with my interest in medical science and exposure to global health whilst interning on Medical Research Council projects in The Gambia, led me to pursue Medicine as a career. Whilst the course is intense, there are already a number of medical students – myself included – starting to get involved with other activities such as research and entrepreneurship. The undergraduate medical course does have time and allocated project space to explore other interests. I plan to do an intercalated BSc in order to enhance my research understanding; ultimately, I aspire undertake a PhD. Though some years away, for my elective I would love to go back to The Gambia. There I hope to apply the skills acquired during my time at medical school and be exposed to situations I may never have come across before (or again!). I believe new challenges and situations are key to furthering personal and professional growth; I hope to discover and maximise these whilst at medical school in order to become a successful and multi-skilled future doctor.

James Frater
Second-year medical student, King's College London

Box 1.2   Postgraduate's perspective

Being a graduate student does offer you greater perspective on the wider professional world that can be put to use during the course. Painfully aware that who you know can be just as important as what you know, I will be keeping an ear out for worthy conferences to attend and look to make contacts wherever possible. I had intended to do some research whilst studying, but due to the intensity of the graduate course it's hard to find an additional 20 hours a month to contribute meaningfully at this stage. I still hope that this may become possible in the later years of the course. I also plan to try and use my elective working at the headquarters of an international research or health body; and at some point beyond qualification, I would like to complete a Diploma in Topical Medicine. I aim to specialise within the NHS but I hope to take the opportunity to live and practice abroad. I have a strong interest in infectious disease and would be keen on a career balancing research with public health interventions. Though, if I am aware of one thing, it is my own ignorance. There will undoubtedly be topics as yet unknown to me that will pique my interest!

Chris Bodimeade
Second-year medical student, Leicester Medical School

CHAPTER 2

Research

CONTENTS

SCIENTIFIC AND CLINICAL RESEARCH

Ashton Barnett-Vanes and Henry D. I. De'Ath

Introduction

Research is central to building the evidence base that advances clinical medicine. As a student, your medical school will aim to expose you to the key research concepts and principles, yet your experience will be limited unless you undertake specific projects or degrees. The aim of this chapter is to introduce you to the fundamentals of scientific and clinical research and signpost opportunities to broaden your exposure and skills.

Scientific method

Basics

Put concisely, the aim of science is to ask questions and draw conclusions. These questions may be aimed at virtually anything, although most will be trying to better understand an issue which is of interest to the scientific and or clinical community – a requirement for obtaining research funding. In medical science, researchers may work on 'basic' or 'preclinical' science issues. The former will usually focus on fundamental concepts utilising investigations in isolated cells or tissue or small species animal models in the laboratory. The latter will have a clinical focus, which, although not yet out of the experimental phase, might be at its advanced stages – with large animal trials or early stage studies with healthy humans. See Box 2.1 for hypothetical examples of basic and preclinical science projects – sample papers are included in the 'Further reading' section at the end of this chapter.

Box 2.1   Example of a basic vs. preclinical science project in brain injury

Basic science: 'This project will examine the effect of xenon gas on isolated neuronal cells harvested from mice. The study will examine changes in the transcriptional activity of anti-apoptotic genes in cells treated with xenon after exposure to mechanical ex-vivo trauma'.

Preclinical science: 'This project will examine the role of xenon gas in preserving motor function in pigs following exposure to a single cortical impact. Once exposed, pigs will be tested for motor skills, speed and dexterity. Typical markers of brain injury will be measured in the circulation throughout the course of the study period'.

Asking questions

Deciding what areas to investigate is an issue for experienced researchers to consider. Laboratory groups are often large and chaotic and have a specific – if somewhat ill-defined – structure (Figure 2.1). In short, you will find professors, senior lecturers, postdoctoral researchers, PhD students, masters/bachelors students and perhaps you – all running around asking scientific questions. Because you cannot speak to cells or tissues or organs or animals, these questions are posed in an alternative way but the concept is the same: cause and (no) effect. For example, to determine whether a cell has died, you can look for a molecule released from the cytoplasm that only leaks out when membranes rupture due to cell death (e.g. lactate dehydrogenase). To check if something has grown, you can count cells. To see if something has been released you can use specific antibodies that give off a colour only if they bind to that substance and measure the intensity of the dye (an enzyme-linked immunosorbent

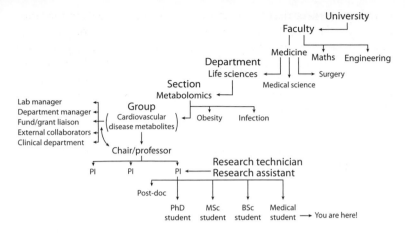

Figure 2.1   Structure of a laboratory group. Note: Principle Investigator (PI).

assay) and so on. Thus, a whole industry now exists full of products, machines and techniques to allow you to interrogate every part of science hitherto discovered.

Realities

While this may (or may not!) sound exciting, it would be disingenuous to not also present some of the realities of science research. While clinical medicine often revolves around patients and advanced clinical investigations (as discussed in the following), medical science projects are often closer to the start of the long and tortuous biomedical pipeline. Thus, there may be few if any patients in sight. Instead, cellular or animal models will be the main experimental vehicles you are involved with. This could mean painstakingly dissecting lymph nodes from a mouse or extracting bone marrow from a rat, without any clear or tangible relationship to the medical ward you have recently grown accustomed to. This is not to everyone's taste; that said, observing and participating in research at the start of a medical science journey offers unique insight into the genesis of medical discovery. In addition, laboratory science (like clinical medicine) is a skill-based vocation, building competence in these techniques takes time and has a steep learning curve. There may also be barriers to your involvement such as licence or ethics hurdles. Check with the lab manager the moment you set foot in the building, as it is their job to ensure the laboratory is compliant with such rules.

Clinical research
Basics

Although the lab is where medical science develops its ideas, the hospital wards and clinics are where they are ultimately applied. Clinical research seeks to improve patient care wherever possible. For example, you might see projects seeking to identify disease risk factors or trial new or more specific diagnosis and treatment methodologies. These might be studies which have originated on the ward or through 'translation' from the laboratory. Either way, as a medical student you are likely to be outside of the decision-making circle, so here is your briefing from us.

Who's who

Clinical research on the ward or in the clinic differs from laboratory research in that it is seldom the only thing clinicians do. Most are practising doctors who commit part of their time to research studies and the rest to delivering patient care; thus, their availability to help supervise or monitor new (medical) 'kids on the block' such as yourself can be very limited. The first thing to do is identify the research team in place, see Table 2.1 for a non-exhaustive list of the usual suspects.

Table 2.1 Typical personnel involved in a clinical research project

Member	Role
Patients (+ relatives)	Give consent to and participate in study
Principle investigator (PI)	Develops and initiates study; obtains funding and ethical clearance; oversees and is ultimately responsible for the research
Investigator(s)	Perform the day-to-day running of the study and most of the research/experiments/data analysis/consent etc.
Research nurse	Manages data collection, educates patients/ staff, obtains consent
Data manager	Codes, enters and manages data including information requests
Medical staff	Manage patient care according to study protocol
Research ethics committee	Determine whether a study is ethical and approve or reject studies based on pre-defined criteria
Research funder/body	Determine quality and suitability of research projects and provide grant funding to those deemed competitive

Process

In stark contrast to laboratory scientific studies where animals are ordered or cells are grown as required, clinical research is entirely dependent on patient recruitment and/or compliance. Clinical studies will often be running a project as part of their routine clinical work; returning to our (fictional) brain injury research example, we can see how this might work as a project (see Box 2.2).

Box 2.2   Example of clinical science project

'A randomised and double-blinded study to investigate if in patients with severe head injury, neurological outcomes at 4 weeks are better if patients are treated in the first 24 hours with a 50:50 mix of xenon and oxygen or the current standard of oxygen alone'.

To perform this study, it needs to first be designed by a principal investigator (PI). It must recruit patients with a severe head injury and must thus be located at an appropriate research site(s). The injury will need to be graded by investigators, likely doctor(s), using a standardised scoring system with predefined study inclusion and exclusion criteria (e.g. no penetrating skull injuries). Next, the consent of the patients or their next of kin will need to be obtained by research nurses and investigators, and if consent is granted, the patients will be randomised. This means that they are randomly assorted into one of the different study groups, rather than a specific predetermined allocation to a particular study arm. Given that the study is examining intervention in the first 24 hours, this sorting will need to be done by investigators and or data managers as soon as possible. After, participants will need to be administered the correct gas, without the patient knowing which they are receiving (single-blind) or the investigator who goes on to score their neurological function (double-blind). All patient demographic data will need to be collected by data managers including age, weight, clinical scores, mechanisms of injury, interventions and so on. Finally, their assessment at 4 weeks will need to be conducted by one or more investigators, preferably maintaining their consistency throughout the study duration. This might be single centre or across whole countries or continents, requiring a phenomenal amount of organisation and communication between PIs and data managers and may last for several years in order to recruit enough patients for the study to be sufficiently 'powered' (valid).

Realities

Thus, given the often slow and steady approach to clinical research, which is always fighting to get enough patients and power, for most of the time, you will not realise any active analysis is happening. Treatment protocols would have been years in the making, and research nurses and data managers will be there to ensure that the process is as seamless as possible. Thus, while in the lab, people can always purpose your empty keen hand; in the clinic, there is not always something immediate for you to do. If you are lucky, you might find large projects in their data analysis phase – here you may have more tangible tasks to work on; however, these may still feel fairly tedious. Figure 2.2 summarises the journey of a hypothetical research study from bench to bedside.

Research at medical school

For those seeking out research opportunities, most medical schools or universities will have a science institute on-site or affiliated with them. Senior doctors may hold positions as clinical science researchers (e.g. academic or lectureship positions) or steer laboratory groups on experimental research related to disease. These groups and individuals are potent resources of information and advice, and you should seek them out at the earliest opportunity.

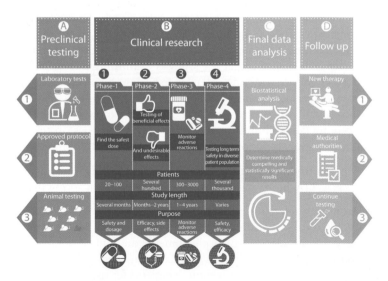

Figure 2.2   From bench to bedside. (Courtesy of Vigyanix.)

Your medical school may also offer you the chance to engage in research more formally, through student-selected projects in a laboratory or clinic or through intercalated degrees or PhDs (covered in Chapter 6). An intercalated degree will offer you the chance to sample research first-hand, usually scientific; however, these projects are often short and relatively basic. A PhD offers true grounding and training in research, but these are an enormous undertaking as discussed elsewhere in this book. Some universities offer science summer schools or placements, where you can approach the supervisors of these courses and offer to visit their lab. Attend lab meetings or events and show yourself to be committed rather than fleeting. When it comes to selecting study projects, see if you can identify your own rather than selecting one off the list.

If you are seeking out clinical research opportunities, gravitate towards centres and departments which are in your areas of interest and ideally with the associated expertise and large volumes of data or patients. Your best selling point to these research teams is your relative permanence. As you will be at medical school for at least 4–6 years, which is longer than most of the doctors on the ward, you can present yourself as a consistent presence over the study duration. However, if you are brought into the team, do not let them down. Have an understanding of your strengths and be honest about what you can and cannot do. If you do well, people will come to rely on you, which can enhance your reputation early as a reliable 'doer'. Quick clinical research opportunities can be carved out in the form of case reports or reviews (as covered elsewhere in this chapter). For case reports, you will need to have a good relationship with senior doctors in your team who can discern what is worthy of writing up. Longer placements and short study modules are good times to undertake a relevant review project with guidance.

Anecdote: Making your own path

When identifying a scientific research project for my intercalated bachelors, I (Ashton) chose to approach a professor working in an interesting field, even though they had not offered a student project to my bachelors course director. I sent them an e-mail and had a discussion. This led to a BSc project which I excelled in. Three years later, I graduated with a PhD in the same supervisor's lab. The lesson? Where possible consider carving out your own path – who knows where it might lead?

Outcomes

As a medical student, the outcomes you can expect from your foray into science are reasonably limited, but not non-existent. It just so happens that some transformational medical discoveries have been made by medical students [1], and many medical students publish papers every year [2]. Publishing is discussed elsewhere in this chapter; however, suffice to say ensure you discuss potential outcomes at the outset of joining a research project or team. Your best chance to publish a science piece as a medical student may be to write a correspondence letter with senior scientists to a recent contentious journal article which may disagree with their own data set. Should you discover something notable in an intercalated degree project, you might find that this data is included as a figure in a larger scientific article – which may warrant your inclusion as a middle author. For a title shot at a high-quality first-author scientific research publication, a PhD is probably your best move. In large-scale clinical research projects, you will probably be a middle author if you are able to participate in part of the study in either data collection or analysis. However, you could lead a review or case report as a first author if done to a high standard. See elsewhere in this chapter for more on publishing.

Anecdote: As one door closes . . .

I (Henry) wrote a review on snake venom which failed to get published, but led to an attachment studying snake venom in the Northern Territories of Australia and spending time in an aboriginal community. This experience in turn was a key factor in being selected to provide medical cover on a BBC expedition in the jungles of South America. Certainly not to everyone's tastes, but it demonstrates that motivation, innovation and enthusiasm can generate fine future opportunities.

Apart from publications, there are ample opportunities to present your research work to student and professional societies and conferences, either nationally or internationally. Alternatively, you may wish to write your work up as an essay for a student competition, many of which come with a sizeable winner's prize and kudos. Try to get something out of your work and, at the very least, request a sign off from your supervisor or a letter confirming participation for your logbook or portfolio.

Conclusion

As a medical student, your opportunity to engage in research is relatively limited unless you undertake specific research projects or further degrees. That said, the quicker and closer you become involved with research in some form, the better, as clinical medicine is not going anywhere without it. Medical school is a relatively safe environment compared to the big scary (and at times scandalous!) world of medical research: bite the bullet and carpe diem – what is the worst that can happen? Good luck, and who knows, perhaps we will be reading about you in a *Science* or *NEJM* issue soon!

Common pitfalls

1. *I am stuck working on a dead end pet project.*

   While most researchers and academics have an eye for a good project, there will occasionally be the clinician who has overrated the relevance or quality of their own work. Avoid lone ranger researchers without any formal group or role and decline to participate in a project you feel has no relevance or potential impact.

2. *I can no longer manage the time commitments of the research.*

   It is common to start out keen and eager, but when exams loom and stresses mount, research can be one of the first things you consider dropping. If you are managing your time well and still feel you cannot handle the extra workload, talk to your research liaison/supervisor and be clear on your commitments. Offer to rejoin once exams are over, but do not be surprised if someone has taken your place when you come back knocking.

3. *Not another histology slide, please.*

   As a junior member of the research team, you are going to invariably get the thankless tasks. Scoring inflammatory infiltrates on 1000 lung histology slides is an unbelievably dull task, but if it will make you an author on the paper and/or you get to write the histology figure – then so be it. At least you will now know what labour lurks behind every paper and glossy figure you see or read in years to come.

4. *I have done more than enough work to be an author, but I cannot see my name on the manuscript draft.*

   See elsewhere in this chapter for publishing troubleshooting.

References

1. Stringer, M. D., and Ahmadi, O. Famous discoveries by medical students. *ANZ J Surg.* 2009;79(12):901–8.

2. Gouda, M. A. et al. Medical undergraduates' contributions to publication output of world's top universities in 2013. *QJM* 2016;109(9):605–11.

Further reading

Barnett-Vanes, A., and De'Ath, H. *Presenting and Publishing as a PhD Student in 'How to Complete a PhD in the Medical and Clinical Sciences'*, 1st Edition. Wiley–Blackwell, Hoboken, NJ, 2017.

Beardsmore, C. *How to Do Your Research Project: A Guide for Students in Medicine and the Health Sciences.* Wiley–Blackwell, Hoboken, NJ, 2013.

Campos-Pires, R. et al. Xenon improves neurologic outcome and reduces secondary injury following trauma in an in vivo model of traumatic brain injury. *Crit Care Med.* 2015;43(1):149–58. (Preclinical science paper)

Dingley, J., Tooley, J., Liu, X., Scull-Brown, E., Elstad, M., Chakkarapani, E., Sabir, H., and Thoresen, M. Xenon ventilation during therapeutic hypothermia in neonatal encephalopathy: A feasibility study. *Pediatrics* 2014;133(5):809–18.

Harris, K., Armstrong, S. P., Campos-Pires, R., Kiru, L., Franks, N. P., and Dickinson, R. Neuroprotection against traumatic brain injury by xenon, but not argon, is mediated by inhibition at the N-methyl-D-aspartate receptor glycine site. *Anesthesiology* 2013;119(5):1137–48. (Basic science paper)

Vigyanix. https://vigyanix.com/.

AUDIT

Henry D. I. De'Ath

Background

Audit is a quality improvement exercise designed to examine current practise against a set standard. While research might ask 'what should we be doing?', audit instead examines 'what are we doing, is it meeting agreed standards, and how can we improve it?'.

Audit is one of the pillars of National Health Service (NHS) clinical governance (Figure 2.3), and audit and quality systems assurance is a requirement of the General Medical Council (GMC) described in their

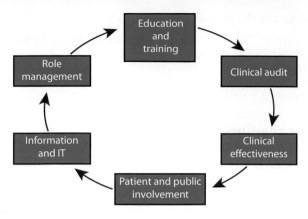

Figure 2.3   Clinical governance cycle.

publication *Good Medical Practice* (2013). At almost every job interview, assessment and placement – someone will direct the word at you
and enquire about your understanding, experience and participation
in the audit process. Given that you cannot avoid it, you might as well
immerse yourself as soon as is feasible. Audit can be generated on any
level from departmental or local, to regional, national or international.

Conducting an audit
Getting started
Foundation/junior doctors are most often involved in the audit process
(and if not should be), so they can be a good port of first call. Failing that,
express an interest with your supervisor during your attachments and
ask to get involved. You are likely to be tasked with collecting data, finding notes or performing some of the more basic (and time-consuming)
components of the process. Nevertheless, such activities should be recognised as audit participation and acknowledged accordingly. They will also
expose you to the process of planning and undertaking such an exercise,
which will prove to be invaluable when it is your turn to lead a project.

Initiating
Audits can either be an analysis of the process, the outcome or the
structure of care. There are a number of steps that you will need to perform in order to undertake a robust project (see Box 2.3). Audit can be
readily planned and executed by junior doctors and medical students
(albeit with some more experienced guidance), and hence, initiative
and autonomy in the process will be both encouraged and admired.

First, make sure the process is registered with the local audit office and keep all these documents as evidence. The audit office can be a great ally, helping you plan and undertake the audit, locate and collect notes and guide you through the process.

Design

An audit, by definition, is against a set standard (a criterion combined with a target), so perform a thorough literature search and establish the criterion you will compare to. The more specific this is, the easier and the better. Refer to national bodies and landmark research papers, hospital trust policies and so on. Design your methods so that they are systematic, reproducible and practical. Consider what data you will collect (define this in advance of starting to collect it) and how you will acquire it. Importantly, determine over what time frame you will amass the data (if prospective) or how long it is likely to take you to acquire it (retrospective). It is worth getting a review of your methods by the audit office or an experienced colleague before starting, as flawed methodology will undermine and undervalue any results. Consider seeking formal audit training through courses prior to starting any project.

Data management

Collect and collate the data and, by all means, invite others to help with this stage. If you identify a deficiency in care or process, develop a simple strategy to overcome this and introduce it into practice. Once your strategy has been implemented, re-audit the process to confirm whether this is functioning adequately and being adhered to. If there are no deficiencies, then no further action is required. Ensure that you keep the data secure and organised. If you have electronic copies of patient notes or data, they may need to be stored on encrypted drives and returned or disposed of in accordance with hospital regulations.

Conclusion

If you finish all the steps mentioned earlier, you will have 'closed the audit loop'. In doing so, you will have determined whether or not your process has led to quality improvement. Thus when you are considering and planning an audit, anticipate the time needed in closing the audit cycle. Failure to do so will be perceived as an incomplete task, so plan your timings accordingly.

Box 2.3   Steps involved in performing an audit

1. Identify the problem or area of inquiry.
2. Search for literature and determine the set standard.
3. Design the audit methodology.
4. Collect the data.
5. Analyse the performance and compare to your set standard.
6. Identify deficiencies.
7. Present and disseminate findings.
8. Implement change to improve practice.
9. Re-collect data and determine effect of change.
10. Sustain improvements.

Output

There are a range of outcomes you can expect from performing an audit. To start, you should anticipate delivering a presentation, usually on a departmental or local level; however, depending on your findings, this could be on a national or international platform too. Publication is rare but feasible if care is improved or you conduct a well-performed project that has interesting results or regional or national implications. Journals such as *BMJ Quality Improvement* [1] are particularly good places to considering publishing an audit. Check also for competitions and prizes available for those conducting audits. For example, in the United Kingdom, the Clinical Audit Support Centre [2] hosts an annual audit competition for junior doctors. At the very least, ensure a sign off on your portfolio and include this on any CV or job application.

Conclusion

Audit is an essential component of improving clinical practice. It is a process that is more readily accessible to medical students and junior doctors than larger-scale research projects, since you do not necessarily need a large team or resources. However, the plaudits that you can expect are also more modest. Start with a feasible project early and drive it to completion before taking on larger-scale audits.

Common pitfalls

1. *Acquiring notes.*

   Acquiring notes is time consuming and sometimes unfeasible and occasionally incurs a cost. This can be highly laborious and can inhibit a successful audit. If you are not convinced the notes are suitably organised or accessible, consider performing a prospective audit.

2. *Insufficient time to conduct audit or complete audit cycle.*

   Plan ahead and be realistic with your time frame. Experienced colleagues can advise on how long you might expect a project to take. Furthermore, be prepared to come in during your free time including when posted to other locations.

3. *Insufficient numbers or data.*

   Perform a pilot study first to ensure the feasibility of your audit, and ensure that you are conducting a project in an appropriate setting. Advertise your audit, and give a presentation before starting, thereby enabling colleagues and medical staff to recruit on your behalf when you are not available. Place posters around and create an area where suitable patient details are left or a pro forma sheet for people to fill when you cannot collect the data yourself.

References

1. BMJ Quality. https://quality.bmj.com/. Accessed on June 14, 2017.

2. Clinical Audit Support Centre. http://www.clinicalauditsupport.com. Accessed on June 14, 2017.

Further reading

Greenhalgh, T. *How to Implement Evidence-Based Healthcare.* Wiley–Blackwell, Hoboken, NJ, 2017.

Healthcare Quality Improvement Partnership. http://www.hqip.org.uk.

Healthcare Quality Quest. http://www.hqq.co.uk.

Tang, C.-M., Qureshi, Z. and Fischbacher, C. *The Unofficial Guide to Medical Research, Audit and Teaching.* Zeshan Qureshi, London, 2015.

The National Institute for Health and Care Excellence (NICE). https://www.nice.org.uk.

WRITING AND PUBLISHING ACADEMIC WORK

**Ashton Barnett-Vanes with Chris McMurran
and Jonathan C. M. Wan**

Introduction

Publishing an academic paper is one of the most significant contributions you can make to the scientific community. As a medical student, many will suggest that this is beyond your pay grade. They are both right and wrong. It is unlikely that you will have the opportunities that could give you data to publish a first-author paper in *Nature* (unless you undertake a research degree – Chapter 6). That said, writing and publishing an article is not beyond your grasp, and certainly, you will have research opportunities that could lead to authorship.

Article armoury

There are several different forms of academic publication. Here, we will focus on those published by journals – books are covered in Chapter 5.

Original research article

This is the most significant of all academic publications, a chance to drive medical or scientific understanding forward into the unknown. They largely follow a set pattern across medical and science journals – Box 2.4.

Box 2.4   Typical research article formula

- Introduction
- Materials and methods
- Results
- Discussion
- Conclusion
- References

The introduction sets the scene for your paper and provides context to your research question. For medical journals, these are seldom more than one page. Materials and methods describe the resources you used in your study and how you performed your investigations. In scientific studies, this will include laboratory reagents and techniques; in clinical studies,

Top tip: Reference formatting

References can be time consuming, particularly if you need to reformat them in order to submit to a different journal. Using a reference management software can significantly reduce the time and stress incurred – many universities and medical schools now offer these to their students. Popular programmes include Refworks, Mendeley, Reference Manager and EndNote. If you are not sure, enquire at your institutional library.

this will include patient selection and procedures. Your results section will describe but *not* interpret your findings. Results are commonly presented as figures – each may have one or more images, and each figure is accompanied by a short legend that describes it succinctly. Figures are referred to in the main result text in detail. Seldom is the literature cited in the results, that is for the discussion.

When discussing your article, the aim is to bring your study and its findings into context within the wider literature. Perhaps you have discovered a finding that goes against previous publications or a novel finding altogether? The discussion will cite the literature in detail, drawing comparisons and contrasts with your own results. You may choose to mention some of the limitations of your study at the end of the discussion. As with the introduction, the discussion of the paper typically extends to no more than a page or two. Finally, the article will conclude with a short summary and a discretionary statement on what needs to be done next. This is followed by a reference list, which must be formatted strictly according to the requirements of the journal.

Letter/correspondence

These are the lowest-hanging fruit of all academic publications, but that does not mean they are not worthwhile. Their purpose is to provide a space for academic debate. This occurs in one of two ways: either as a critique of another research article, which is short (~300 words), or as short opinions or sharing of miniresearch findings on a topical issue (~400–600 words). Usually, between three to five authors can be included. Increasingly fewer journals accept letters, but the major medical journals still do. Some high-profile medical science journals accept research letters, but these are more like concise original articles and not to be confused with a typical letter to the editor. Writing a letter will hone your academic writing skills and give you a taste of the journal system. Try using a student-selected or elective project as a chance to drum up sufficient perspective or data to submit a letter.

Comment/essay/perspective

These are a longer essays or opinions which bring a certain perspective or wisdom to the reader. Although they are not out of a medical student's purview, many journals will expect these articles to be authored by experts. That said, if the comment or essay pertains to medical education or another area you feel well qualified in, perhaps you can make the case for your suitability.

Review

The purpose of a review is to improve the understanding of a medical and scientific topic. This could be through a qualitative synthesising of existing research coupled with a splashing of your own wisdom and insight (a narrative review) or by careful assessment of the literature based upon predefined criteria (a systematic review). Narrative reviews are typically written by experts to be authoritative; systematic reviews should in theory be more accessible for junior academics like yourself to conduct. There is not enough space to cover the details of writing a review – see [1] for further details. Briefly, a systematic review will need to define clearly what issue you are seeking to review and a set of search criteria to follow. You and your colleagues will then scan perhaps hundreds or even thousands of papers that meet this criteria to check if they are actually relevant. The point here is to capture as much information as possible and then whittle it down. Narrative reviews are considered slightly more biased, given that no or few criteria may be used. With your selected papers, you will then summarise their findings, draw conclusions and perhaps make further recommendations. Systematic reviews are usually done alongside original research projects.

Academic publishing: Ins and outs

Now that you are aware of the different ways by which you may publish, how exactly do you go about it and end up on PubMed?

Authors

Article publishing is increasingly a collaborative exercise. Gone are the days of one or two people publishing large-scale studies. Today, anywhere between 5 and 20 authors may be on a research paper. As authorship is a coveted title which confers academic success and/or promotion, there are strict guidelines governing who can be listed as an author [2]. Often, you will be involved in research led by senior doctors or researchers. However, if you have led the work – you should be the first author. If you have contributed substantially to someone else's project, you should be a co-author. The two most sought after positions on a paper are the first ('did the work') and last ('designed/funded the work') author slots.

As a medical student, you could be tempted or even put under duress to include senior doctors or academics on the work you have done. Alternatively, you could find yourself being pushed down the author list on account of your junior standing. Both of these should be resisted. While it is common to have senior authors who may do less of the leg work than yourself on a paper, they must have done serious critical review or made creative contributions. Including someone as an author who has done nothing on the article is both unprofessional and unethical. If you are in doubt, speak to the person responsible for research standards or ethics at your institution.

Journals

Journals are the portal that transports your work to the wider academic community. They are revered and heralded in grand rounds and laboratories the world over. But beyond the glitz is a simple fact: journals are a business. They require funding to survive and that is fuelled by article fees, donations and advertising money. The value of the latter is heavily influenced by its readership and circulation in print and online. Thus, journals want to publish things which attract attention and garner interest. Added to this mix is a desire to publish material which is relevant and impactful in the field. Such articles are likely to be referred to more often in other papers or cited, and these citations generate a metric by which journals can be ranked by: the so-called impact factor. There is therefore a temptation for journals to publish material which shows a positive result and not things which show little or no change – even if that may still hold wider significance – a phenomenon called publication bias. Finally, journals are included in different indexes which makes them easier to find and which has become a marker of their perceived quality. Thus, journals which are indexed in PubMed are considered more favourable to submit to. Journals want to become indexed and have to meet a set of criteria in order to do so.

Authors want to publish material in PubMed indexed journals with a high-impact factor, which are considered more reputable, for two reasons: these journals are more visible to readers and authors get more prestige or academic points for publishing in them. Thus, if you are co-authoring an article and tasked with choosing which journal to submit to – you may find yourself scanning a list of PubMed indexed journals ranked according to impact factor. While this approach is understandable, check that the journal is relevant to your article by looking at the kind of papers they publish. Each journal has its own identity and niche, a good senior author will be able to give guidance on where – and where not – to submit.

Submissions

Submitting an article is both exciting and laborious. These days, submissions are almost always processed online and via e-mail. Although most authors still go ahead and submit directly, more journals now offer a *pre-submission enquiry*. This gives you the chance to pique the interest of the editor, before spending hours jumping their electronic submission hoops. If you are ready to submit for real, you will need to format the manuscript appropriately, build image files of all your figures (if necessary) and write a short covering letter to the editor. Guidance for all these steps is included on the journal website as 'author instructions'. Study these and triple-check that your submission conforms to them; journals have no problem returning a submission (repeatedly!) which does not meet their guidelines – see Box 2.5 for the common items to include.

Box 2.5   Ingredients for a successful submission

1. Covering letter
2. Manuscript (+ title page)
3. Tables and panels
4. Figures
5. Author statement form
6. Declarations and conflicts of interest
7. Completed protocols and checklists

Once you have successfully submitted, there will be a delay as the journal considers your manuscript. If they feel that it is not suitable for publication in their journal, it will be rejected. If your submission *could* be suitable, it will probably be sent out for peer review. This is where one or more other academics in the field examine your article and decide whether it merits publication as it is (rare), requires further revisions (common) or should be rejected (also common). Editors will usually follow the advice of the reviewers. Some articles, such as letters or comments, may not be peer-reviewed, and it will be at the discretion of the editors to accept or reject. Getting a decision from journals can be an extremely slow process. While the top medical journals have a faster turnaround, most journals could take 2–6 months to make a decision on your article. If a rejection decision is returned, you can appeal to the editor if you are not happy with the review. But usually, their decision is final. If the reviewer asks for revisions, complete these carefully and return them as soon as possible. This usually involves providing a clean and track-changed copy of your manuscript, as well as including all changes and your own responses in a bullet-pointed list in a new covering letter. Your article may also undergo statistical review if you have included any statistical data.

Anecdote: Appealing a reviewer's rejection

When submitting a paper from my PhD to a journal, I received a couple of pages' worth of reviewers' comments. I duly addressed these point by point, and after a further few rounds of revisions received, to my surprise, a rejection from the reviewer/journal. Disappointed, I e-mailed the editor to make clear the concerns they may have had were unnecessary and provided all the details at my disposal. I was invited to resubmit a final revision and the paper was accepted two days later: never give up.

Publishing

If you have your paper accepted, congratulations! This will go through copy-editing and typesetting by the journal, and you will be required to process any author or open-access fees. Your institution might be able to assist you in covering some or all these. If submitting from a country with lower income, fees may be waved. And often, fees are waved for students, irrespective of country of origin. Once the paper has been edited, you will receive a proof. This must be checked and any issues responded to urgently. It is common courtesy to share the proof with your co-authors. Often, journals want these returned within 24–48 hours. Once returned, your paper may first appear rapidly online as a *corrected proof*. Eventually, it will be assigned to a journal issue and appear in print or online for all to see and read happily thereafter.

Case study: Running a medical student journal
Chris McMurran and Jonathan C. M. Wan

To advance medical care, clinicians must not only just perform research but also communicate this effectively with their peers and the public. Student medical journals, such as the *Cambridge Medical Journal (CMJ)*, which we edit, focus on publishing medical students' work, often giving them their first experience of the review process. This offers students the chance to get recognition for medical school projects, audits and essays that may otherwise go unpublished. It also helps students develop their skills in academic writing as a stepping stone for future endeavours.

WHY EDIT?

Having a go at editing gives you a look behind the scenes of academic publishing. It is a unique opportunity to develop your critical appraisal skills: what exactly distinguishes a really good manuscript? These skills are a valuable asset in any clinical career, not least when self-critiquing your own work. Apart from editing, it is also a chance to try running a website, learn the tricks of social media and have fun in the process!

IN A NUTSHELL, HOW DOES IT WORK?

Taking the *CMJ* as an example, our three editors manage the journal, website and publicity and have overall responsibility for articles coming through. We also have a number of section editors who coordinate the peer review process between reviewers and authors (Figure 2.4). Reviewers are generally academics and consultants in Cambridge, although we sometimes cast a wider net if the field is particularly specialist. Our target audience is United Kingdom-based medical students, but we have found that increasingly, students and doctors in other countries have submitted work.

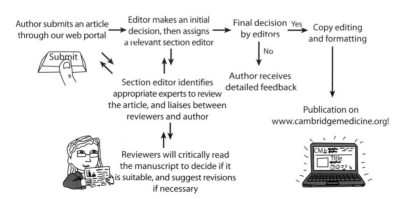

Figure 2.4   Running a student medical journal.

DID IT HELP YOU MAKE THE MOST OF MEDICAL SCHOOL?

Editing for the *CMJ* has been a rewarding way to learn some useful skills ranging from critical appraisal to hypertext markup language coding to tactful communication of feedback. Part of the fun has been the interesting challenges it has thrown us: dealing with authors that do not take criticism well or making the final call on a controversial article. With good team work, you can run a journal to be proud of without cutting into too much free time.

HOW CAN I GET INVOLVED?

To start up your own journal, think about what would make it unique – why should people submit to you over other journals? It is important to develop a pipeline for the submissions process and try to build up a bank of reviewers. Online platforms such as Scholastica (https://www.scholasticahq.com) are custom made for administrating a journal and have made our lives much easier. Feel free to get in touch if you have any questions – and happy editing!

Conclusion

Writing and publishing an academic paper is an art which takes years of practice. It remains the age-old medium of communication between researchers and practitioners. However, there is no reason why this training cannot begin in medical school. Try your hand at correspondences to get a feel for the writing and submission process. If you find yourself working on a larger project, leading or assisting others, volunteer to write up a first draft and build your experience. If you really enjoy the process, consider editing for a journal. Publishing papers, like most worthy endeavours, is a trying process littered with rejections. And while it might not be Broadway, seeing your published name up on the screen or in print will warm the cockles and show that it was all worthwhile.

Common pitfalls

1. *Where do I find an opportunity to publish?*

    Publishing academic articles requires intellectual work. You may be able to do this without much research when writing opinion articles. However, research articles will require you to be involved in a research project. Look out for opportunities on student-selected projects and intercalated degrees; alternatively, approach senior doctors in your medical school and enquire whether they need an extra pair of hands on data analysis or writing. Show yourself to be competent and reliable – and let the good times roll.

2. *I keep getting rejections from journals.*

   Journals can be a fussy bunch. But remember, you are likely to be biased in your assessment of the quality of your work. It takes experience to know what type of paper a journal will publish. Either you are aiming at the wrong journal or the work is of insufficient quality or significance. Consult with senior colleagues; if you are convinced the work merits publication – keep submitting.

3. *'I want I want I want I want me me me me now now now now.'**

   While publishing is an enjoyable and positively reinforcing activity, some medical students and junior doctors can go overboard. Venting paper after paper of low-quality work purely to saturate PubMed does not achieve much, and your good-quality work may be lost in the crowd. Resist the temptation to illogically chop your research into several fragmented articles – focus on quality papers which make a valuable contribution to the literature and hope someone will actually read them.

References

1. Hall, G. *How to Write a Paper*, 5th Edition. Wiley–Blackwell, Hoboken, NJ. Accessed on June 10, 2017.

2. International Committee of Medical Journal Editors. http://www.icmje.org/. Accessed on June 10, 2017.

Further reading

Albert, T. *Winning the Publications Game: The Smart Way to Write Your Paper and Get It Published*, 4th Edition. CRC Press, Boca Raton, FL, 2016.

Barnett-Vanes, A., and De'Ath, H. *Presenting and Publishing as a PhD Student in 'How to Complete a PhD in the Medical and Clinical Sciences'*, 1st Edition. Wiley–Blackwell, Hoboken, NJ, 2017.

Cambridge Medicine Journal. http://www.cambridgemedicine.org/. Accessed October 17, 2017.

---

* Adapted from the 1991 motion picture *Hook*.

CHAPTER 3

Organising and leading

CONTENTS

ESTABLISHING A GROUP OR CAMPAIGN

Ashton Barnett-Vanes

Background

Tackling issues, whether they be simple or complex, acute or chronic, tractable or seemingly intractable, requires patience, determination and *teamwork*. This chapter will introduce you to establishing a group and running a campaign. It offers a basic introduction from a student's perspective, there are a great wealth of organisational texts and guides out there for richer detail.

Another group?

Wherever you see groups, coalitions, organisations, societies and so on (herein collectively termed *group*), you invariably also find confusingly titled committees, steering panels and 'presidents'. While it is perhaps human nature to build bureaucracy, life as a medical student is complicated enough already. Thus, choosing to establish a group or organisation should be a decision reached after long consultation and ideally evidenced by clear objectives and aims. It is not for me nor anyone to say what is or is not a worthy cause; however, your team's motivation and public/donor support rest on it – so choose well. Examples could be a peer–peer support network to promote student mental health, raising awareness of the lack of essential medicines in under-served populations or campaigning for equitable access to health training.

Getting started

Box 3.1   Key details for establishing a group

1. Board or committee
2. Objective, aims and mission statement
3. Constitution and by-laws
4. Strategic plan
5. Company registration or incorporation (if applicable)
6. Website, e-mail and social media presence

The board or committee of your group will need a clear division of labour, with roles and responsibilities included in the constitution. A sensible and preferably uncomplicated leadership structure is also required. Roles and titles can vary enormously, common examples include chair/president, deputy/vice, treasurer, secretary/communications, webmaster and advisors. The key areas to cover with these roles (which may overlap as required) are an external-facing individual to engage with external stakeholders, someone to maintain the fluid functioning of the internal team, a member who can operate social media/e-mail account(s) of the group, and someone capable of building and maintaining websites. From there, any number of operational members can be involved working on one or multiple projects.

A mission statement outlines in a few short sentences why your group exists and what it aims to do and supplements the concise objectives and aims. The constitution and by-laws are documents detailing the governance of your group – they provide information on how common issues are to be handled such as membership, financial handling, leadership change or group dissolution. They are also integral to its wider credibility in the eyes of the public, prospective members and donors. A strategic plan will outline short-, medium- and long-term approaches to achieving your group's objective and will usually flesh out the mechanisms by which it intends to do this. Should you be handling finances during your operations, you may choose to register your group as a company or charity/non-profit. While beyond the remit of this chapter and book, such activities

Table 3.1 Helpful online resources for a group

Website builder	Business email client
https://www.wix.com/	https://gsuite.google.com
https://github.com/	https://products.office.com/en-au/business /office-365-business
https://wordpress.com/	https://sso.godaddy.com/
Social media	**Fundraising platform**
http://twitter.com/	http://kickstarter.com/
http://facebook.com/	https://www.indiegogo.com/
https://pinterest.com/	https://www.rockethub.com/
https://www.youtube.com/	https://www.gofundme.com/
http://linkedin.com/	https://www.crowdcube.com
Collaborative file sharing	**Conference call/communications**
https://www.dropbox.com	https://hangouts.google.com/
https://www.google.com/drive	https://www.skype.com/en/
https://onedrive.live.com/	
https://spideroak.com	

thrust you from student campus advocacy into the legal world of accounts, annual returns and taxes. Seek professional assistance/ support from the get-go including consulting an accountant or financial advisor. Finally, few groups will survive long without the life force of the World Wide Web and all its trappings. Table 3.1 details common go-to resources for those looking to establish an online presence.

Engaging with stakeholders

Stakeholder is one of these terrifically vague and business-like terms. When I first heard it, I thought – where/what is the stake? It is loosely defined as all the people/groups involved in your project. Say you are trying to get the cost of a drug lowered – stakeholders would include the pharmaceutical manufacturer, the health systems who purchase it, doctors who use it and patients who are intended to benefit from it. There will also be other non-governmental organisations (NGOs) or governments who want it cheaper (or not) and so on. When building your group or campaign, you will need to start engaging with these individuals or institutions, and this can be quite an art.

Start by building up a group of allies early – senior individuals, societies or organisations who believe in your cause and are willing to give you a covering letter or introduction when needed or a testimonial for your website, for example. Economy starts at home, so look at your own medical school, university and city/region for potential supporters. It is common courtesy to keep these partners abreast of your progress, every 6 months should suffice and never send anything out with their name on it before asking them (or their secretary) to sign it off. Approaching donors is covered elsewhere in this chapter and in Chapter 7. As for large institutions whom you wish to influence or support – be patient and keep trying. You may be able to secure a meeting with their leadership, in which case make your questions clear and offer ways to support them. You might find yourself knocking on a closed door and ignored for years. If so, look for moments when leadership changes occur to reintroduce yourself and impress your cause onto their successors. However, this works both ways, and seemingly cooperative staff can be replaced by those who are less/not interested or heaven forbid – hostile.

Getting things done
Activity
Medical students may use the groups they join or establish for myriad activities. When considering yours, make sure that you justify how each activity adds to/supports your overall objective. You may wish to begin by doing some research that highlights the issue(s) you wish to address. Publishing this in a peer-reviewed journal not only brings you a much wider audience, but also strengthens the credibility of your group by showing that reviewers and editors recognise both the issue and your ability to produce a high-quality piece of work. If research is not easy to achieve, you might use an awareness campaign involving online and face-to-face techniques to bring the issue to the attention of your constituents or the wider public. Ideas could include an e-mail mailshot advertising a public meeting or a large one-day or two-day event bringing a range of people and stakeholders together (see 'Organising an event: The conference' section). See Box 3.2 for examples of activities for getting your message to a wider audience and stimulating action.

Box 3.2   Getting your message out

- Word of mouth
    - ✓ Do not underestimate the power of speaking to someone about an issue.
    - ✗ Scalability and message control are drawbacks.
- Leafleting
    - ✓ A well-designed leaflet can catch attention and convey key facts.
    - ✗ Leaflets have a tendency to end up rapidly in the bin; offset this by putting a scannable QR code on your leaflet directing readers to a website/digital resource.
- Blog
    - ✓ A blog is a rapid way to convey information to a potentially wide audience.
    - ✗ A blog can have a short half-life and thus require your own social media momentum; busy blogs will add new content all the time, pushing your piece further down the list.
- Published article
    - ✓ A published article gives you peer-reviewed authority and gets your message out in perpetuity to an educated audience.
    - ✗ Publishing an article is a slow process and must be journal specific; if it is not published open access, few members of the public may be able to read it.
- Media
    - ✓ Established print or TV media outlets offer you the chance to reach thousands or millions of readers/viewers quickly.
    - ✗ Expect to work to close deadlines; be cautious of how your project is interpreted or presented.
- 'Twitter storm'
    - ✓ A Twitter storm can help raise awareness and involve large numbers of people each contributing a modest effort, e.g. a retweet or hashtag.
    - ✗ Twitter is a closed audience; hashtags come and go and you will likely be eclipsed by the trending *catdoesmoonwalk*.
- Video/advert/documentary
    - ✓ Catches attention, engages audiences and can drive your message home innovatively.

> ✗ Requires large amounts of planning, production and editing; it is often costly; a poor-quality product can bring down your whole campaign.
> - Crowdfunding
>   - ✓ Crowdfunding is an eye-catching medium to raise awareness and generate funds; platforms often let you upload a range of content and media.
>   - ✗ Crowdfunding is a high-intensity project that needs nearly full-time input to be successful; several high-profile platforms operate an all-or-nothing strategy, which means you *have* to meet your target to get any money.
> - Public meeting/festival/conference
>   - ✓ An interactive way to engage with hundreds or thousands of people to advance your cause.
>   - ✗ It is a large-scale project that takes months to years of planning and execution.

Anecdote: Running a campaign, one step at a time

After completing an internship at the World Health Organization (WHO) in 2012, I worked with a group of former interns to tackle a long-standing issue of inequitable representation of interns from developing countries. We realised that without strong research behind us, we would fail to catch people's attention given the size and reach of WHO. We set up a group and published research in several journals, including the *Lancet Global Health*, *UN Special* and *BMJ Global Health*. This offered us a solid foundation on which to campaign. We used blogs, adverts, videos, documentaries, crowdfunding platforms and face-to-face meetings to raise awareness and stimulate action. In 2016, several WHO member states raised their concerns at the World Health Assembly necessitating responses from WHO. The lesson was to patiently build a foundation that was credible before raising the profile and employing a range of campaign techniques.

Fundraising

Whatever impact you are seeking to make, soon enough, you are going to need funding to sustain your group. Where possible, using university resources (e.g. printing, desk space) is advisable as it is likely to be cheap or free. However, if you are looking to attend a meeting in a different country or produce a documentary on your cause, for example, obtaining funding is a necessity (unless you are willing and able to self-fund). For a new group or campaign, you are unlikely to have the background or resources to immediately obtain grants from the Bill & Melinda Gates Foundation. That said, medical students and junior doctors have previously set up groups in partnership with universities and societies to successfully obtain such funding – so where there's a will there's a way. Your best bet to get substantive funding relatively quickly is through contributions from interested donors or organisations, who ideally you can get introduced to; from institutional grants (check your local university or student societies); and via crowdfunding. Table 3.1 contains details of common crowdfunding websites – each has its own requirements and criteria so check them in advance before committing/announcing anything public.

Impact

Measuring impact is an essential skill. In medicine, this is routine: Are the vital signs improving? Is the C-reactive protein coming down? And so on. In campaigns and group action, this is not necessarily as easy, but it is the key metric on which observers and donors will gauge your success. Simple measures could be how many members joined, your current revenue, number of cake sales and so on. Other measures could be number of publications, events organised or sponsored, policy changes in your area of action, public statements by key stakeholders and so on. Whatever they are, it is essential that you document them regularly and share them on your website and with key stakeholders such as members, supporters, donors and the public. Good opportunities could be annual reviews or reports from organisations which have detailed information you can measure and compare to previous years. For example, in the WHO Internship Programme project as discussed earlier, I would scour the WHO Human Resources Annual Report for the latest statistics on internship participation: were things improving, getting worse or staying the same? This was essential information to inform our onward work.

Sustainability

They say all good things come to an end. This may be true, but it can be vigorously offset by a well-planned handover. If you do not want your project to end when you leave, advertise for and identify a team that can replace you. You could linger on as chair or senior advisor to ensure that things do not fall off track; if you have established major

sponsorship or funding support from donors, this may be a requirement of theirs. Either way, a clear constitution, strategic plan and
objectives should offer your comrades a clear path to both follow and
develop as they take over the reins. If you feel that your group has
achieved its goals, there is nothing wrong with folding it and exiting
stage left. If you choose to do so, make sure you dissolve as per your
constitution, and if you have a legal standing or financial obligations,
make sure these are fulfilled accordingly.

Conclusion

Establishing a group or running a campaign is an endeavour that takes
much thought and patience. Often, worthy causes take years if not
decades to make real impact – so what are you waiting for? Building an
effective team is paramount. Good governance and oversight reduces
the likelihood of problems and makes those that do arise easier to
solve. Successfully running a group or campaign shows true leadership qualities, and who knows where it might lead!

Common pitfalls

1. *Forgetting you still have a career ahead of you.*

    It is easy to get absorbed in a campaign, especially if it is par-
    ticularly contentious or fast moving. However, remember to stay
    professional. Getting arrested outside an embassy might look great
    on Twitter but not necessarily in front of your medical school dean
    or future employers.

2. *All talk, no action.*

    A challenge for student groups and activists is translating their
    well-founded concerns/frustrations into tangible outcomes. This is
    as much an ethical or moral discussion as it is a practical one. Try
    to aim for activities that make a real difference, however small –
    rather than activities that make those involved in it feel better but
    do nothing on the ground.

3. *Not knowing when to say goodbye.*

    It is easy to get comfortable running a certain group or cam-
    paign. After a couple of years, there is a risk your fresh blood and
    enthusiasm has congealed and become the slow and bureaucratic
    machine you had initially hoped to disrupt. Always look for fresh
    talent to come in and challenge your ideas and methods. And if you
    feel that it is time to hand over the reins, do so.

Further reading

Example documents from the WHO Internship Programme Campaign:

Barnett-Vanes, A., Feng, C., Jamnejad, M., and Jun, J. Towards an equitable internship programme at WHO: Is reform nigh? *BMJ Global Health* 2016;1:e000088. doi:10.1136/bmjgh-2016-000088. http://gh.bmj.com/content /1/2/e000088.

Barnett-Vanes, A., Kedia, T., and Anyangwe, S. Equitable access to global health internships: Insights and strategies at WHO Headquarters. *Lancet Global Health.* 2014;2(5):e257–9. http://www.thelancet.com/journals/langlo /article/PIIS2214-109X(14)70211-6/fulltext; https://www.kickstarter.com/project s/1529563606/304477200?token=4695b2a6; https://www.youtube.com/watch ?v=Y9uT8X7k2Oo&feature=youtu.be.

Fletcher, T. *Naked Diplomacy.* William Collins, New York. 2016. [An interesting discussion on the changing role and methods of modern diplomacy. A useful read for those seeking to engage and influence in the digital age.]

Hochschild, A. *Bury the Chains.* Macmillan, New York. 2005. [A terrifically inspiring book on what multifaceted cross-generational advocacy and campaigning looks like and without internet, smartphones or the computer.]

Kahneman, D. *Thinking, Fast and Slow.* Penguin Books, London. 2012. [An international bestseller on thinking and decision-making.]

ORGANISING AN EVENT: THE CONFERENCE

Ruben V. C. Buijs

Background

As introduced in the previous chapter, medical school offers the opportunity to participate in and demonstrate organisational leadership. One of the high-profile situations you may encounter is *the event*. Throughout your career, you will attend receptions, awaydays, conferences etc. Organising one of these is an opportunity to shape the agenda and achieve an outcome which may have an impact on hundreds if not thousands of people. This chapter uses organising a conference as a vehicle to explore the steps involved in running an event from a student's perspective. It is hoped that the experiences contained in this chapter equip you with both insight and a plan that can be applied to any event you decide to lead.

Building and leading a team

Chairperson

Your first task is to appoint a chairperson. This person will be the external-facing leader of the conference. They need to be charismatic, determined and committed to the cause. They will get the plaudits if it is a success and, equally, will be most tarnished should the conference fail. Previous experience leading a group or conference is desirable – and it is absolutely essential that they are a good communicator.

Core committee

Once you have found your chairperson, it is now time to build the rest of your team. Start with peers, other medical students with credentials that suggest willpower, discipline, experience in organisations or an overall sense of good work ethic. You are best off interviewing them; this not only gives you the chance to explore their qualities face to face, but also demonstrates the professionalism and transparency of your conference from the outset. At the interviews, you will want the conference organiser and chairperson present. However, you may also wish to include a third party who has nothing to do with the conference – and can thus provide a more objective assessment of whether the candidate is well suited for the job rather than the team per se. When choosing your team, try to maintain some balance in demographics and personalities. In the interview, make sure to add a few questions that they will not see coming to gauge how they respond under pressure. See Box 3.3 for a list of common roles and responsibilities and Figure 3.1 for how they all fit together.

Box 3.3   Example of a conference-organising team

Core team
- *Chairperson:* The face and voice of the board and is responsible for all outcomes and maintains cohesion in the committee
- *Secretary/vice chairperson:* Organises the agenda and locations, keeps minutes and manages the props required for each meeting

- *Treasurer:* Drafts budgetary plan, arranges financial support and keeps track of all spending and income

Additional positions

- *Logistics director:* Organises the venue, catering and social programme; drafts up the playbook; and is the boss during the actual conference
- *Scientific programme director:* Drafts up the scientific programme, leads the abstract selection for poster and oral sessions, contacts potential keynotes and maintains communications with them
- *External communications director:* Spreads the word to all potential attendees through universities, social media, associations, (non-)governmental organisations and individuals
- *Design director:* Manages the website and promotional material and produces all creative content, such as newsletters, posters and logo

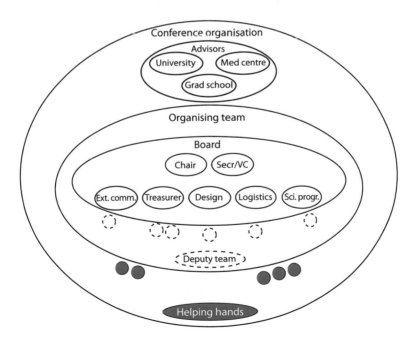

Figure 3.1 Conference team.

Gelling the team

Once your team has been assembled, the chances are that none of the members know each other well. Dedicate a large portion of the first meeting to getting to know one another. While socialising is important, there is work to be done besides your already-demanding medical studies, so combine leisure and labour as much as possible. This can be accomplished by alternating between 100% formal meetings and 80%/20% formal to social gatherings every few meetings. Lastly, it is highly recommended to have a weekend away with the team as the conference approaches. This not only helps gel the team, but also gives people the chance to have a good argument and release any tensions. If animosity persists, restructure tasks so members will not collide; failing that, ask someone to leave – your first priority is to deliver a high-quality event, not keep everyone happy.

Name and date

Whatever the topic of your conference, you should be able to write it down in one sentence. Often, conferences are named after medical associations or a specific field, but these do not always make the contents or aims clearer. Develop a two- to three-line official statement that encapsulates the aims, incorporating factors such as novelty, cause and future impact. Ensure that you are clear and have agreed on your primary and secondary audiences. Next, choose a date or at least a season in which you hope to organise the conference. In many cases, the date will be similar to that of previous years. Diverging too much from this period will require justification and may dissuade longtime attendees from coming. Make sure you decide early on and stick to it, as you want to send out the announcement of your conference as soon as possible.

Content management

Two forms of content should be managed: scientific and social. The scientific content of a conference must be administered by a dedicated individual and is generally structured as follows: invited keynotes, oral/poster presentations based on submitted abstracts and a social event. This can be expanded upon in many ways. Keynotes could be invited to moderate discussion panels; parallel workshops with a limited amount of attendees can be organised; and semiformal networking sessions, such as scientific speed dating, can also be featured.

Keynote speakers

The keynote sessions and oral presentations are the main events for attendees, so these need to be ironclad before more risqué elements are introduced. Like the lineups for music festivals – if you recognise the bands, you are more likely to go, right? The search for keynotes should be started as soon as the general goals for the conference are decided upon. The scientific programme manager will need to sell the conference to the potential keynote. So what will your conference bring the speaker? A sizeable and enthusiastic public is the minimum requirement. Some organisations may be able to pay a lot of money for the speaker, but most keynotes will only require a modest alignment with their ambitions or interests (and their expenses covered) in order to take your proposition seriously.

Speakers can be found all over the place. It is easiest to find local experts from your own university or other national universities. But an international cast is most likely to catch the attention of attendees and sponsors. Start e-mailing Nobel prize winners, high-ranking journal editors and directors of renowned hospitals or research institutions. As long as you can sell why they would be interested in your conference, you can contact anyone you want. You risk nothing and could end up with a very inviting lineup – see Box 3.4 for a typical keynote invitation e-mail.

Box 3.4   Example of invitation letter for a high-profile keynote speaker

Dear Professor/Dr/etc. [. . .],

Firstly, may I congratulate you on your ongoing success with [. . .]? We believe that your impressive career, current position as [role] of the [department] and outstanding contributions to medical science are a true inspiration to the young and ambitious medical professionals of the future. Therefore, on behalf of the board of the [conference name], I cordially invite you to be a keynote speaker at our conference to be held on [date] at [venue] in [city, country].

Our conference is [history and relevance of the conference]. For the first time since [inaugural conference], our city of [. . .] is honoured to be hosting, and the conference will be attended by approximately [50–100–500–1000] [types of delegates, e.g. students, trainees] attendees from [all over the world, the United Kingdom, Europe etc.]. With this conference, we aim to [. . .]. The slogan of this year's conference is '[. . .]'.

We would be honoured to welcome you at our conference and have you deliver a keynote lecture about [. . .].

If you decide to attend our conference, we will finance your entire trip and stay in our beautiful city.

For more information, please visit our website [. . .]. If you have any questions, please do not hesitate to contact me.

Thank you for considering our request. We hope you will honour us by accepting our invitation.

Yours sincerely,

Abstracts

Abstract-based oral and poster presentations depend on the quality of your audience. Assuming that the quality of submitted abstracts is normally distributed, there will always be a top 5–10% of abstracts that outperforms the rest. Ideally, those will be selected to speak. The next 40% should be eligible for a poster presentation and the rest should, ideally, not make the cut.

Abstract selection should be performed diligently, preferably by individuals qualified to assess the quality of a study or a researcher, based on the abstract. The scientific content manager is responsible for the method of abstract analysis, which should be transparent and standardised (e.g. common scoring system, internal validation of scores).

Logistics

Venue

Where the conference is held is of major importance. The shorter the distance between your sessions and workshops, the better. One might choose (or be forced) to have multiple venues necessitating some unwanted transiting; this is also true for the location of arranged lunches, coffee breaks and other informal components. However much you try, your attendees *will* get lost, so it is imperative that you diminish this risk from the outset. Have an abundance of directions lying around, directional arrows or posters and a good map for everyone in their delegate bag or on their phone (see later).

Marketing

Once your keynote lineup is clear, your public relations (PR) officer can start spreading the word and making sure that people hear of your conference as soon as possible. Sponsors will react positively to an intriguing keynote cast, even if you do not have any attendees yet. As the abstracts start rolling in, you can provide a better estimation of the number of attendees you will have.

Delegate registrations

Handling registrations can be an arduous task for beginners, but if you have experience with database research, you may feel quite at home. The secretary or another well-suited committee member will need to prepare a spreadsheet database containing all the variables you wish to collect from your attendees (see Box 3.5 for examples).

Box 3.5   Delegate details

- Surname, first name
- Role at the conference (attendee, keynote, workshop host etc.)
- Country/city of origin
- Field of interest
- Hotel preference (which hotel, single or double room, breakfast included etc.)
- Workshop preference (in case of limited availability)
- Payment received and registration complete?

If you choose to administer delegate registration via your conference website, make sure you collect all necessary details on the registration page; it is worthwhile using automated messages to inform the attendees of their registration/confirmation. Have a dedicated committee member collect and organise these messages on a daily or weekly basis, depending on the frequency of registrations.

Accommodation

Depending on the audience of your conference, there are a couple of options to research for housing your guests. In the case of a younger (med) student population, it is possible to arrange housing at the dorms or apartments of volunteering colleagues and fellow students. This helps lower the price of your tickets, but will also make for less reliable quality management and will entail additional micromanagement in pairing people based on gender or preferences etc. Hotels and hostels are the next best option, and often, larger hotel chains are willing to negotiate on accommodation fees if you are able to maximise their occupancy rate for a given number of nights.

Try securing one or more of the following deals:

1. Lower prices for every 25 or 50 that may attend.
2. Pre-determined price for a certain estimated number of guests. If you are 90% certain that over 200 guests will stay, you could book 200 rooms in advance for the discounted price.
3. An extensive cancellation period, in case your primary estimate is wrong. Some hotels offer full restitution for cancellations 2 months in advance or 75% restitutions if you cancel in the final 2 weeks before the event. Negotiate for what suits you best.
4. Offer international hotel chains a sponsorship deal, lowering the price for ad space at your conference. If you have a returning conference, you could offer to accommodate your guests for the coming 3 years in one of the chain's hotels.

Events and catering

Despite the banality of coffee breaks and conference lunches, this is where you as organisers can still make a difference. Bad memories will linger longer and stronger than good ones, so make sure terrible food or insufficient coffee cups are not among them! On the other hand, organising a flashy dinner on one or more of the conference days will definitely have a lasting impact. Just like selecting your keynote speakers, think outside the box (specifically Box 3.6). Don't forget to have a tasting session with the caterer first.

Box 3.6   Fun conference activities

- Dine at a special location, e.g. a fancy restaurant in an old building or on a boat.
- Combine dining with scientific speed dating or prize ceremonies.
- Invite magicians or musicians for pre- or post-dinner entertainment.
- Organise a tasting event involving local delicacies.
- Instead of renting your own venue with a band or DJ, make use of your local bars and clubs and have your fellow committee members guide the conference attendees all over town.

Prizes/awards

Your visitors may never admit to it, but winning best oral presentation or best poster is on their minds. Having a prize that may well win back their investment (i.e. conference ticket, travel expenses or hotel accommodation) will draw attention. Try to think of something quirky and memorable. Handing out a couple thousand pounds/dollars/euros in cash is difficult, since money for your conference can be hard to come by. You also risk frustrating other delegates by having their conference fees ending up in the pockets of their fellow visitors. Linking your awards to your sponsors is an effective method of making sure the prizes are something special.

Conference app

A web or smartphone app dedicated to your conference can be very helpful in providing easily accessible information and will leave a great lasting impression. Most conferences have a booklet with all the conference info, pictures and summaries of keynotes and attendees and advert space. This can also be done in an app, for a similar price, saving paper and giving you more data to work with. Most companies have fully formed example apps to peruse. Get a quote and then haggle, fill your app up with the necessary information and decide on the ad space for your sponsors. Thus, even if the app costs more than a paper booklet, you could get your money back with a bit of tactical sponsor placement.

Approaching sponsors, donors or partners

The treasurer of a conference has a tough job – this task is generally most removed from the professional experience of any medical student or doctor. Not only do the funds need to be raised with gusto, they must also be kept safe. Delegating an assistant to help the treasurer is a prudent move, particularly during the preparatory phase.

Pitch

The fundraising manager will first and foremost be working with people. Most mid- to large-sized institutions have particular employees in place for such PR-related tasks – so what do you have to sell? Some potential perks for sponsors or partners are summarised in Box 3.7.

Box 3.7   Your conference selling points

- *Your target audience*: Either in size or in degree of importance.
- *Your keynotes*: Big shots in any field attract money, simple as that.
- *Venue*: What if you have your conference in Strasbourg or Brussels, near the European Parliament? Or what if your venue is bound to some high-tech clinic or technology? Do not underestimate the value of being known for something by association.
- *Your message, vision or aims*: Perhaps your conference is on a subspecialty that has garnered a lot of attention lately, and the sponsor provides services specifically to that field.
- *Big (social) media presence*: Whether your conference will have many attendees or not, if you have a well-visited website or Facebook page, you will have the raw data to back up that the sponsor will be well advertised.
- *On-site presentations*: On-site presentations of donors/ sponsors/partners.

Running the conference on the day

In the weeks preceding the conference, you should be meeting up with your committee members more frequently to discuss the minute-by-minute playbook and confirm all the tasks of each committee member. In this preparatory phase, the chairperson and logistics manager must speak with every individual about the playbook activities for each day.

On the day itself, the chairperson no longer reigns supreme as they will need to give the opening speech, be present at every talk, have a chat with the keynotes if appropriate and maintain a presence for the audience. All other members, however, have delegated responsibilities for the daily logistics – and the logistics manager is their leader. All communications will be relayed through this manager, who is always up to date on what is going on. For this reason, the manager has no tasks other than making sure every step of the playbook goes as planned. The other members should have both a task and a primary station (see Box 3.8 for examples). Some places must have a continuous presence such as the reception where keynote speakers, sponsors and the lost and confused will present themselves.

Box 3.8   Key locations/stations of a conference

- *Registration booth*: At the opening of the conference, man the registration booth with as many as you can spare. Afterwards, always have two members stationed here for keynotes, late arrivals, sponsors etc.
- *Sponsors/partners*: Dedicate one member to visit the sponsors every break to chat and make sure they're comfortable.
- *Lecture halls*:
  - Outside: Before every session, have one or two members show the entrance to the lecture halls. They will go inside and close the doors behind the last guest.
  - Inside: At the start of the lecture, make sure it is clear who is responsible for providing the microphone and a glass of water to the keynote and who is running around with a mic for audience questions. Also, prepare one or two committee members to ask questions when no one in the audience does so.
- *Workshops/poster sessions*: Depending on the amount of poster/workshop sessions and the exact locations, it is optimal to assign one member to guide each small group of attendees to the respective locations and to bring them back to the main hall afterwards.
- *Dinner/social events venue*: One hour to 30 minutes before your social event starts, have one committee member stationed there to check if everything is going as planned. If possible, have the same member stand at the door to personally welcome all arriving guests at the venue.

Outcomes: After the conference

It is not over yet. With hopefully a successful conference under your belt, there are still a couple more things to finish. Prepare a thank you e-mail and send it to attendees, keynotes, committee members and auxiliary figures a couple of days after the conference ends. This is also a good chance to do a post-conference survey to gauge the opinion of attendees. If you had a photographer or a film crew at your event, inform delegates of when they can expect the pictures and films to appear on the website. Lastly, if a new conference is already in the making, let your attendees know the details in consultation with the

Top tips: T-minus 1 week to 1 hour

One week or days before the conference:

1. Determine the proper etiquette.
   a. Do not use your phone if you are not calling your fellow committee members.
   b. Do not run or raise your voice in the public areas.
   c. Smile a lot. This is your day. If things do get too much to handle, notify the logistics manager and retreat to the break room.
   d. Complaining is for the day after.

Evening before:

2. Go out dining with all committee members and helping hands. Lift the spirits, take some pictures and go to bed early.

One hour before the opening:

3. Final meeting at the selected resting hub. Discuss final questions and go over the most important tasks.
4. Synchronise your watches.
5. Make sure your telephones are fully charged.

new organisers. To ensure the event can be repeated in subsequent years, some form of information transfer to the next organisers will be needed. Have all the committee members draft up a short timetable of their actions during the year and note a couple of pitfalls, challenges and helpful tips that you ran into. Share helpful feedback from your survey too.

Now, it is finally time to relax. Have a break, update your résumé and LinkedIn page and be proud of your accomplishment. You have earned it. Then get back to your studies, there is an exam you need to pass next week!

Conclusion

With the information in this chapter, you should be able to construct a plan towards making your conference or similar event a reality. While this chapter is condensed, I hope it gives you a sufficient heads-up on the key caveats of event organising. Needless to say, you will need to draw on your own creativity and critical thinking throughout the process; attracting committee members with some degree of experience will definitely help. Finally, do not forget what you are doing this for. It may be a hobby, another valuable addition to your social life or a way to take your mind off the drudgery of medical school, but it should be, although irredeemably cliché, plain and simple fun.

Common pitfalls

1. *What if the number of submissions is too low?*

   If the number of attendees is too low, this will harm the conference financially, not only in attendance income but also by deterring sponsors. Yet, if the quality of the content is inadequate, future conferences will be harder to advertise to previous attendees and sponsors. Whatever you decide to do (e.g. extending submission deadlines or reducing the number of sessions), be aware of the fallout and try to limit the damage as much as possible.

2. *Signs of non-commitment in your team.*

   This can weigh heavy on the entire team and great care must be taken to immediately discuss issues when they arise. Most problems relate to time management and deadlines and can be handled through swift and open conversation about what the issue is and assigning the right and willing person to help out.

3. *Burnout.*

   Your physical and mental health and university performance are the priority. All the committee members will need to vow to look after each other, but it is the final responsibility of the chairperson to make sure all tasks are divided equally or at least appropriate to the capacities of each member.

4. *CREAM: Cash rules everything around me.*

   Money is going to be an issue no matter how well the organisation is going. You will always need more. Therefore, make sure you have a pre-determined and rational budgetary plan and sponsorship goal. If you are constantly being turned down by sponsors, it is most important to keep going and not lose hope.

Further reading

Collins, J. *Good to Great: Why Some Companies Make the Leap . . . and Others Don't*. Harper Business, New York. 2001. [This book is about companies and may go beyond the scope of the work you will be doing, but essentially, the author discusses the core tenets of effectively meeting your goals in making your conference/company great.]

Gawande, A. *The Checklist Manifesto: How to Get Things Right.* Metropolitan Books, New York. 2009. [Surgeon and writer Atul Gawande has written multiple must-read books for medical students and laypeople alike, but this one specifically aids anyone working towards important endpoints and where mistakes are costly.]

Chapter 4

Writing and speaking

CONTENTS

PUBLISHING A BOOK

Ashton Barnett-Vanes

Introduction

Writing a book is a considerable endeavour to undertake at any time in one's life; deciding to write one during medical school is not for the faint-hearted. A book is intended to be a lasting contribution to the literature, with a half-life much longer than an original research paper. Further, unlike academic papers, which are typically unpaid, publishing a book is an academic activity that may lead to *some* financial remuneration for the editor/author. This is without doubt a bonus but should not be the driving factor in your decision; I wouldn't want to know my hourly rate based on the time invested, and I doubt i'm alone. Writing a book will bring you into contact with stakeholders you may have seldom interacted with before: commissioning editors, copyeditors, marketing officers, lawyers, trade unions and so on. This should be seen as an exciting opportunity, but you are now a small fish in a great lake – flap with caution. With whole *books* written on this topic, the purpose of this section is to bring you up to speed on the process and provide a strategy along four key steps: conception, pitch, preparation and publishing.

Conception
Any ideas?

Originality is key to publishing, be it a book or an academic paper. The market you are targeting and the publishers that serve it are looking for new material. Thus, in choosing to write a book, you really ought to have a good idea. Given that you are going through medical school, it is likely that your idea will be influenced by this environment. Medicine, health and education are common themes in books written by medical students, although the romantic novel is not out of your grasp too, if so inclined. Perhaps you want to write a new textbook of anatomy or you think your mind maps should be everyone's? Whatever the idea, as soon as you have one, it needs stress testing. Your first question should be – will this actually work? There are a range of mediums to convey information, a book is only one of them. Blogs, journal series, videos, apps and so on are all effective ways to disseminate your wisdom. Are you sure a book would be the best way to get your message across?

If you are convinced it is, the next step is to do your research. Has anyone done this before? Is there anything similar in your country or elsewhere? What about in the other mediums mentioned earlier? If there is an identical book already published, it is going to be difficult to convince a publisher of the case for your idea, there may also be legitimate copyright concerns. The other two scenarios are your idea is – to the best of your knowledge – unique and unpublished or there is another book(s) that partly crosses onto the territory of yours. This latter scenario is common, given the crowding that pervades most niche markets, but you should be wary of pitching something that has been done *ad nauseam*: do we really need another book on 'getting into medical school'?

Development

Once you have stress-tested your idea and are convinced that it has not been already done, it's time to develop it. The first question is who is your audience? For example, national or international; students or educators; medical or non-medical. What form will it take – a solo effort or a multicontributor piece? Will it fit into your back pocket or need hoisting up as a full-colour illustrated atlas? These details are not only critical for the pitch, but will also shape the way you develop the book beforehand. If you are going to author it solo, are you qualified and what experience can you draw upon? Likewise, if it is going to have several contributors, do you know who they might be?

Once you are clear on the basics, it is time to work on the details. You will need a title, a provisional table of contents (ToC) and a list of potential contributors if applicable. It is also worth drafting a chapter or two, to see if your ideas actually translate well onto the page. Armed with these materials, your next move is getting some informal feedback. Perhaps there are academics in your university that have edited or published books. Find them and ask for their advice. Likewise, if your audience are first-year healthcare students, ask them to read through your chapter. Does it make sense? Would they use it? And importantly, would they *buy* it?

Pitch

If you have come through these hurdles and you are still convinced that you are on to a winner – it is time to get pitching. By now, you should have an idea that is new and would make a good book, a clear view on its presentation and knowledge of your target audience.

Finding a publisher

This chapter will focus on publishing through a professional publisher, for details on self-publishing see towards the end of this chapter. There are myriad publishers, houses, imprints, groups etc. Navigating them is a challenge, particularly given your likely relative inexperience. While you can laboriously browse their websites, a simple way to start narrowing down which publishers to target is to look for similar titles already published – you may already have these details from when you researched the competition. Scour the high-street or online bookstores for comparable titles and collate a list of the publisher names and dates. Go to the website of each publisher and compile a list of the commissioning editors responsible for the field of your book.

Building a pitch

Once you know which publishers you are targeting, you need to browse the pitching instructions for each. While these will differ somewhat, they typically follow a common pattern; see Box 4.1.

Your author information will need to include a CV and previously published material. The title of the book and abstract are self-explanatory; ensure that your abstract does not overhype the book as the commissioners will be looking for the ToC to come up with the goods. The target audience can be subdivided: e.g. primary (medical students), secondary (other healthcare students), tertiary (medical educators).

Box 4.1   Common pitch content

---

1. Author information
2. Book overview (title + abstract)
3. Target audience
4. Provisional table of contents (ToC)
5. Example chapter
6. Market information
7. Competing titles
8. Other details (word count, delivery timetable etc.)

The ToC should be detailed, ensure that your chapters flow logically and are sufficiently differentiated. Include your best example chapter, there is no convention on which to include. While many opt for the introduction, there is a strong argument to include a chapter which is actually at work in educating/informing the reader rather than introducing them to the book. The market information you provide will be central to the publisher's calculation of its perceived profitability. Be as detailed as you can and get hard statistics if possible.

Anecdote: Market information

When pitching my first book to Wiley–Blackwell, I contacted the United Kingdom's National Statistics Authority to enquire how many PhD students were registered in the United Kingdom for each subject. I included this information in the pitch. Not only did this provide the commissioning editors with the latest figures, but it demonstrated my commitment to the project and attention to detail. The pitch was successful.

You will need to be thorough in your research on competing titles, there is nothing more embarrassing than missing one of the books that the publisher you are pitching to has on their shelf. Include the title, authors/editors, publisher and International Standard Book Number (ISBN) and provide a succinct summary of each competitor title. Somewhere in the pitch, you will be asked to explain why your book differs from the competing titles; be concise, clear and courteous in distinguishing your book from the crowd. Finally, be realistic in word counts and delivery times. Six months to one year is a reasonable lead time between commissioning and book submission.

Review

With your pitch prepared and submitted, you will be hoping that it goes out for review (if it does not, see common pitfalls at the end). This gives you and the publishers the chance to test the views of members of the target audience you have identified. Review can take anywhere between 2 and 6 months and will be provided to you along with a tentative decision from the commissioning editor. If successful, you will be given the outline of an agreement. If the reviews have come back recommending edits, you will need to make adjustments in consultation with the commissioning editor with the potential for further review. If the reviews recommend rejection of the concept, see common pitfalls. Reviews that come back positive may also provide some feedback to incorporate into the book. This is helpful; however, you are entitled to disagree with these suggestions if you feel that they go against your vision for the book. Ready to sign on the dotted line?

Preparation

Until now, much of your work has been provisional – promises rather than reality. Now that you have an agreement, the real work begins.

Contract

Depending on the kind of book you are writing, you and other coeditors/authors will agree to a contract with the publisher. This is a legal document, with legal implications. Notwithstanding the medical lawyers among us, you are strongly advised to seek outside support in assessing the merits of the contract.

All contracts will differ in style and scope, but there are several common themes. Your responsibilities as an editor/author will be spelled out, and you will be liable for breaching them. All material in the book must be original or have copyright permissions if obtained from elsewhere. Publishers will have different rules on how to edit and proof the manuscript. Some will expect you to index the book – a serious undertaking [1]; others will do the indexing themselves. The rules for publication will cover anything from the free copies you/contributors are entitled to, to the cover and style of the book and what say you have over it.

Royalties and accounting are, for many, the most significant clause of the contract. You are strongly advised to seek outside support from professionals; remember, the contract will be seeking to profit the publisher as much as possible. Many author groups and societies offer

---

Box 4.2   Common contract content

1. Editor/author responsibilities
2. Permissions
3. Copy-editing, proofs and index
4. Publication
5. Royalties and accounting
6. Copyright and intellectual property
7. Revisions and new editions
8. Warranties and indemnity
9. Termination

---

free or paid contract vetting to ensure the deal you are getting is reasonable. For example, in the United Kingdom, the Society of Authors offers a free contract-vetting service if you are an annual fee-paying member. Royalties will include detailed provisions on the monies you are entitled to before or after discounts, tax and shipping deductions. Attention to detail on the wording is critical. You may also wish to include a clause that allows you to inspect the publisher's accounts pertaining to your book. Finally, you may be offered or request an advance for the book. This is a lump sum of money (~£250–£500 for a first author) which the publisher usually gets back by taking it off your royalties. Advances are becoming rarer but you should still ask for one.

Alongside financial considerations, the contract will ask you to hand over copyright and intellectual property – effectively, your idea is now the property of the publisher. This will have an impact on your future works which may be of significant likeness to the current project. Future revisions and editions are self-explanatory, but pay attention to the wording of the clause – will you be given full autonomy to select coeditors/contributors? Indemnity and warranty covers who picks up the bill if something goes wrong – e.g. if you fail to get a permission and the publisher gets sued: call your bank, quick. Termination governs the responsibilities of you and the publisher, which, if broken, may constitute grounds for ending the contract. For example, if the publisher does not pay you or, after 5 years, you still have not submitted the book.

Finally, note that if you are editing a multicontributor book, contributors will also need to sign a contract. These are usually simpler and denote their responsibilities and what benefits they get, e.g. royalties (rare) or free copies of books (more common). While they are signing the contract, you as editor/author are ultimately responsible for the delivery of the project, as referred to, e.g. in Clause 5.1, page 8, section c, paragraph 7, lines 418–422.

Writing

With the contract signed, it is time to get cracking. If it is just you writing, what are you waiting for? If you are editing a multicontributor book, you will need to do a considerable amount of organising:

1. Contact or confirm with contributors their willingness to participate.
2. Provide them with example materials (ToC, sample chapter), clear instructions on the content of the chapter and a first draft deadline.
3. Follow up with them periodically (not incessantly) to check on progress; always be polite and responsive in answering their queries.
4. Be gentle with their drafts, if it requires revision, be guiding and supportive – do not eviscerate it with track changes (initially).
5. Ensure that they have signed their contract and collect their current details/affiliations for the book.
6. If you are both happy with the draft final chapter – keep them periodically updated on how the book is coming along and when they can expect to receive their free hard-copy.

Anecdote: Contributor tension

When editing a different book, I wanted two contributors to co-author each chapter. This innovatively synthesised two perspectives and viewpoints to cover all the angles for the reader. However, while most chapters were plain sailing, some contributors experienced a difficult – if albeit relatively short – engagement. In one case, the differences between the co-authors were so irreconcilable, I had to merge their two sections myself. The lesson: think about the compatibility of contributors if you are asking them to work together on a chapter.

If you are editing, your role is to ensure that the content is complete and there is a continuity of flow and style across the chapters. This is a significant undertaking. Contributors bring a breadth of experience and insight but will have different writing styles – and varying opinions on your edits too!

Manuscript

With all the chapters in and vetted, your work does not stop. You now need to produce a manuscript. This will include everything: final ToC, foreword, list of contributors and affiliations, chapters and the index. During this process, you should get support from the copy-editor/ author liaison officer who will provide you with guidance on how they wish the manuscript to be presented. This will ensure a seamless transition from computer document to bookshelf. Word processors, such as Microsoft Word or LaTeX have helpful functions to make this easier, including ways to standardise your headings and automatically generate ToCs and built-in indexing tools. The better job you do of this now, the less hassle down the line when dealing with copy editor queries and proofs. Once you are happy with the manuscript and confident that it meets the publisher's expectations, submit it already!

Publishing

With your new fame and fortune in press, it is tempting to start looking for that tropical island you can soon retire to. But before you do. . . .

Proofs

Proofs will come back from the publisher and you will have a relatively short period to return them, perhaps only a month or two. Remember, as per your contract, publishers will likely have the right to edit for house style, which means words changing, the letter Z appearing in places it should not and so on. You may also wish to share the proofs of each chapter with the contributors, particularly if you feel that the changes are significant. Either way, if you do not respond to the proofs, contract permitting, they can be published without your approval, so take them seriously. If you have serious issues with the content or layout, communicate this as quickly as possible together with reasonable suggestions on how to address them. Ensure that you are happy with the front/back cover and check that all names and affiliations are correct.

Launch

With your book now published, you should congratulate yourself and all those who were part of it. A team curry or some other event could be called for. To drum up publicity and sales, you may consider a book launch. This could be done in partnership with a society, university or institution and the publisher. It gives a chance for you to lap up praise, but more importantly, ensures that the book is made visible to the target audience you plotted about all those months/years ago.

Self-publishing

Self-publishing your work offers you benefits and drawbacks [2]. You skip the elongated pitching and approval stage and can get straight to developing your book and getting it out there. Publishers often subcontract their work to freelancer proofreaders, copy-editors and so on. There is nothing stopping you from doing this directly and cutting out the middle man if you have the financial means to do so. Further, the marketing budgets of publishers are not what they were, and thus, self-promotion is increasingly key to drive sales and publicity for non-established authors – whether they self-publish or not. Finally, you are likely to make more money from your sales; self-publishing websites and companies offer you anywhere up to 50% of sales – see Box 4.3 for further details. However, self-publishing comes with risks. If you are not well-known or a start-out author, cutting through the crowded space of self-published work can be challenging. A respected publisher confers credibility onto you and your title. Publishers offer you critical appraisal and inside knowledge on crafting your book and targeting your market. If not from them, can anyone else offer you this support? If successful as a self-publisher, you might choose to approach (or be approached by) a publisher to take on the marketing and revisions of your book in the future.

Conclusion

Writing a book is a demanding endeavour; however, the rewards are many. Not only do you have your name and work on show for others to benefit from, you may actually earn a little too. Liaising with contributors can be taxing, but is more than offset by the win–win when the book is in everyone's hand. It can take 2+ years from idea to *Amazon* – good luck!

Box 4.3   Popular self-publishing channels

- Lulu (http://www.lulu.com)
- MagCloud (http://www.magcloud.com/)
- iUniverse (http://www.iuniverse.com/)
- CreateSpace (https://www.createspace.com/)
- Dog Ear Publishing (https://www.dogearpublishing.net/)

Common pitfalls

1. *My pitch has been rejected – what should I do?*

   This is a common issue faced by academics. The key question is whether it is you or them? Are you sure your idea is suitable for a book and has not been done already? If so, check that you have managed to convey this successfully in the pitch and get another experienced pair of eyes to look over it. If you are convinced that it is them, go down your list of publishers and keep trying, incorporating any feedback you get in the process. Rejection is said to be a necessary test of character.

2. *Show me the money.*

   The returns you get on a piece of work which you have invested such time and effort in are small for unestablished authors. It is quite common to receive somewhere in the region of 5–10% of royalties on sales. You can and by all means should try to negotiate this; seeking support from experts is strongly advised. However, be prepared for little or no budge. That said, if you don't ask, you don't get.

3. *My contributor has gone AWOL.*

   Writing a book is a bit like driving a bus. Some contributors arrive on time with their drafts, others take repeated nudging (or extortion), and some may literally never turn up at all. Stay calm and work on getting a replacement. Liaise with the publisher too if you are approaching deadline. While it can feel disappointing, try not to take it personally – things can crop up that make once doable commitments, such as chapter writing, undoable.

4. *Indexing my book is painful – help.*

   Nobody said it was going to be easy. If your publisher does not do indexing for you, try using built-in services in your word processor to speed things up [1]. Alternatively, you can contract a professional indexer, but you will need to pay for this – which could end up writing off a few years' worth of royalties. If you are going through hell, just keep going.

References

1. *Guidelines for the Preparation of an Index.* http://www.ugapress.org/upload/indexing.pdf. Accessed on June 14, 2017.

2. Friedman, J. Start here: How to self-publish your book. Jane Friedman. 2015. https://janefriedman.com/self-publish-your-book/. Accessed on June 14, 2017.

Further reading

Sutherland, A., Nelmes, A. and Kaye, P. How to write a medical book. *BMJ Careers*. 2013. See http://careers.bmj.com/careers/advice/How_to_write _a_medical_book.

WRITING AND BLOGGING

Adam Staten

Introduction

At its best, medicine is a collaborative endeavour that relies on the free flow of ideas and knowledge. There are now more opportunities than ever for people within healthcare to share these opinions and to have them challenged and finessed through open discussion with colleagues from around the world. Writing, either in print or online, is a fantastic way to air your ideas and engage with the wider medical community in order to achieve this.

Why write?

There is a simple pleasure in seeing your words in print and knowing that your contemporaries are paying attention to them. But there are other more tangible benefits to be gained from writing and blogging.

Debates and connections

A well-written article or blog post can gain an enormous audience. If there is an issue about which you are passionate, then there are few better ways to get your message out into the public consciousness. Chat forums and journal correspondence mean that you can discuss your message with an international audience, start a campaign to publicise it and gain the attention of people with the authority to influence the outcomes. Writing gives you the opportunity to engage with the medical community and to create connections within it. A well-written and thoughtful article can prompt responses from people who would like you to speak at events, join committees, have more articles commissioned or collaborate on research.

Job prospects and money

If nothing else, blogging and writing will score bonus points on your CV. You may not always be adding significantly to the weight of medical knowledge, but writing shows that you are thinking about issues within healthcare and that you take an interest in the thoughts and research of others. Without doubt, this makes you stand out from the crowd against whom you will have to compete throughout your medical career. Sadly, there is not a great deal of money to be made from writing or blogging within medicine. Plenty of people are keen to write and this makes it a buyer's market with editors holding the purse strings. Having said that, there are a few opportunities to earn small amounts of money by writing and this can help ease the financial strains of being a medical student.

Opportunities and outlets

There are myriad websites, journals, blogs, newspapers and chat forums that are all hungry for contributors. Each of these platforms has its own benefits and drawbacks, and these should be weighed to help you decide where you want to submit your work.

Academic journals

Academic journals can seem like formidable institutions, but the people who edit them, and the people who read them, are interested in a breadth of opinion on matters that concern their area of interest. They are therefore keen to hear the voices of colleagues at all levels of seniority and training.

As discussed in Chapter 2, the bulk of a journal will usually be filled with research, but many journals feature opinion pieces, letters of response, book reviews and articles detailing interesting and unusual experiences. These are all good subject matter for medical students. Be thoughtful as to what the readers of the journal might be interested in reading about. For example, if the health service is struggling to attract people into gastroenterology, consider writing an article about what it is that attracts you to or puts you off a career in gastroenterology. This is the sort of thing that the editors will want to know and that only medical students can give a grassroots perspective on. Printed journals offer the satisfaction of seeing your writing preserved for posterity in hard copy, and all articles within a journal, whether it is groundbreaking research or a letter to the editor, are awarded a CV-boosting citable reference.

Blogs

Most major journals will have a big online presence including a blog. Submitting posts to a blog is often less intimidating than submitting to a print journal, and the submission criteria are usually less stringent. Importantly, the publication process is usually very quick. In contrast to a journal, which may take months, the lag time of a blog is usually just a few days. This means you can write about things that are current and see almost immediately whether people agree with you or not.

Besides the blogs associated with academic journals, there are thousands of blogs concerning health matters, many of which are open to outside contributors. A well-written article will develop a momentum of its own once shared on social media, even if the blog is relatively obscure. The intelligent use of social networking platforms can get your work read by tens of thousands of people in a matter of hours in a way that is simply not possible in a printed journal. Finally, there is no reason why you have to submit your work to someone else's blog. If you feel that you have lots to say and do not want to be subjected to anyone else's agenda, there are numerous platforms that allow you to host your own blog. This may not give you the warm sense of pre-acceptance that comes from having your thoughts published on a widely recognised outlet, but it does give you complete editorial freedom over the content.

Mainstream media

Opportunities within the mainstream press are harder to come by. Most regional and national publications will have a medical correspondent on staff who will provide commentary on the hot health topics of the day. However, if you have a unique and interesting view on a news story, there is no reason why you should not seek the wider audience that newspapers and magazines offer. This is a great way to have your thoughts read by thousands of people but be prepared for rejection, or more likely, non-response. In the case of success, be prepared to provide your work on a tight deadline.

Website content

There are various opportunities, almost invariably online, to make a little money from writing. The public appetite for information about health and lifestyle issues is insatiable, so the internet is full of websites in search of content. The knowledge you have as a medical student, and your ability to assimilate and understand new knowledge from recent research, is not to be underestimated.

Many websites are desperate for credible writers to provide content and will often provide a small fee for doing so. If you feel that you could explain the physiological benefits of a Mediterranean diet in a way that the public will understand, then you have a gift that may earn you a little pocket money. However, beware of bogus websites or those asking you to provide content on commercial products with no evidence base etc.

Anecdote: Think international

There is no reason to feel constrained by geography when looking for work as a writer. There are numerous websites on which people in need of writers advertise. As long as you can write in the desired language, then consider an application. In the past, I have picked up a little extra cash writing content for an Australian lifestyle website, writing articles for an American medical social network and editing translations of Polish research papers. Often, the fact that you are approaching a topic from the viewpoint of a different country can enable your work to appear more unusual and thought-provoking to readers based elsewhere.

Getting started

For those interested in writing, it can be difficult to know where to start. Rejection is commonplace, and it can be disheartening, but with writing as with so much else, success begets success. Everything you write is something to put in your portfolio and another experience you can mention when pitching for and submitting further work.

Think big, start small

Aspiring writers find themselves in a catch-22: editors are looking for experienced writers, but how do you get experience if no one will publish you? You can start gathering experience by writing for publications where there is no expectation of experience. University and medical school blogs, for example, or even national student blogs, such as the *British Medical Journal* student blog, are written by students for students. With a few articles under your belt for this type of publication, you become a much more attractive prospect to other publications. See Figure 4.1 for an example hierarchy of common outlets.

Mainstream media

Writing in the mainstream media is largely reserved for writers higher up the food chain, but there are opportunities for new writers. For example, the *Huffington Post* is an American based news website with a huge, international audience that invites bloggers from

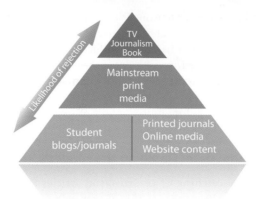

Figure 4.1   Common writing and blogging outlets.

all backgrounds. In the United Kingdom, *The Guardian* is a major national newspaper that supports a widely read blog specifically created to give a voice to healthcare professionals (*Views from the NHS Frontline*). Although uncommon, if you stay alert, such outlets present an opportunity to get your work published in the mainstream media.

Commissioned work

If you are adaptable and able to produce work quickly, then paid work is not hard to come by. For example, Upwork.com is an online forum where freelance writers writing in any genre, in any language and with any level of experience can find work. Here, you can find all kinds of jobs from writing patient information leaflets to books. This is also a good place to find work writing for health and lifestyle websites. Similarly, the *European Medical Writers Association*, which is even more international than it sounds, is an organisation through which you can find work in medical journalism as well as work writing for the pharmaceutical and biomedical industries.

How to write a blog post

Blogs are by nature topical, informal and conversational. They are an opportunity for you to express your personal opinion and, as such, are often personality driven. You should therefore write in whatever style that comes naturally to you. Successful medical blogs often give a personal perspective on big, topical issues and frequently make use of anecdote and individual experience to ground complex issues in the real world. They are also an arena in which people can express opinions that are outside the mainstream. Web editors often like the blog to have an element of controversy because this tends to inspire debate and response, resulting in increased traffic on the website. While balance is to be encouraged, most bloggers write their articles in order to put a point across. Good blogs make a case for their author's point of view and invite it to be challenged and debated. See the articles by Stec [1] and Brenner [2] for advice on how to structure a blog post.

Anecdote: Catching the reader's eye

Blogs need eye-catching or controversial articles to attract attention. When the *British Journal of General Practice* launched its blog, I submitted a ridiculous article about how I considered a particular item of clothing to be a red flag sign for depression. It was well received and generated a lot of traffic for the new blog. I am sure the blog, now well established and much more serious in tone, would not accept a similar article today but, at the time, it suited the editor's purpose.

Pitching and submitting

There are many people who want to see their writing in print, and editors working for any type of publication are usually swamped with enquiries and submissions. It is easy for your work to get lost in the crowd if you fail to pitch it well.

Audience and agenda

It is absolutely essential to work out what the audience of your chosen outlet is. Read through previous articles of your chosen publication and work out what type of articles they normally publish; only pitch your article if you believe it fits with the general ethos of the publication. Note that all media outlets have an agenda. This may be straightforward; for example, it is safe to assume that a diabetes journal is likely to have the agenda of sharing knowledge about diabetes, but, particularly with respect to more mainstream media, the real agenda may be political, moral or economic.

Follow the guidelines

Find out what the submission guidelines are for the publication. They are almost always listed on the website but, if you cannot find them, send a brief e-mail to the editor enquiring if they accept unsolicited submissions and ask how they like the work to be submitted. Once you have found out what the guidelines are, follow them to the letter. Editors will have little or no patience with a submission that does not conform to them.

Keep your CV up to date and consider tailoring it to appeal to different types of publications. For example, include more detail about academic achievements if you are submitting to an academic publication and perhaps more detail about lifestyle and extracurricular activities if you are pitching to a health and lifestyle website. Above all, when submitting and pitching, remember that if you do not ask, you do not get. There is never any harm in a speculative submission or approaching a publication. The worst outcome is that they say no and you have lost nothing but a few minutes of your time.

Conclusion

Writing can be incredibly rewarding at both a personal and a professional level. There are numerous ways in which you can get your thoughts out into the world and, by doing so, have a chance to entertain, challenge and influence your colleagues and the wider public. If you feel that you have something important to say, then you should write it down and try to get people to read it, there is nothing to lose in the attempt and there may be much to gain.

Common pitfalls

1. *Never ever use patient identifiable information.*

   This is a sure way of nipping your medical career in the bud before it ever gets started. You may think that no one will recognise that

Top tips

1. *Keep it short.*

   Most blog posts or articles are around 600 words in length. Readers will quickly lose interest in articles much longer than this, so be savage when editing and cut out anything that is off topic.

2. *Use social media.*

   If you want people to read what you have written, then share it. Articles can take on a life of their own once they are out on social media no matter how obscure the original platform on which they are published.

3. *Respond to comments.*

   Blogs and articles should be about starting a conversation, but the conversation quickly dies if the main participant falls silent. Engaging in the conversation your article begins can be the most rewarding part of writing, as, after all, one of the main reasons we write is to share ideas.

4. *Be thick skinned.*

   The world of writing can be one of endless rejection, and the world of blogging can be one of irate rebuttal. People may respond to your blogs rudely, aggressively and ignorantly, but try not to take offence – it is all part of the fun!

photo of a fungal toenail infection, but the patient will, and they may be very unhappy to have had it splashed across the World Wide Web.

2. *Do not quote erroneous or fabricated data.*

No matter where your writing appears, remember that you are writing in the guise of a future medical professional, and as such, your writing should stand up to close scrutiny. Inaccurate data will rob you and your opinions of their credibility. Ensure editors and commissioners are clear on your background from the outset.

3. *Do not be rude or offensive.*

No matter how tempting it may be to get drawn into an aggressive argument, remember that whatever you write is out in the world forever, and ill-judged comments can haunt you in unimagined ways years down the line.

References

1. Stec, C. The anatomy of a perfect blog post (Infographic). *Hubspot*. Hubspot, Inc., Cambridge, MA. https://blog.hubspot.com/marketing/anatomy-perfect-blog-post. 2016. Accessed on June 14, 2017.

2. Brenner, M. Anatomy of the perfect blog post. *Marketing Insider Group*. https://marketinginsidergroup.com/content-marketing/anatomy-of-the-perfect-blog-post/. 2015. Accessed on June 14, 2017.

Further reading

Medical writing. ABPI Careers. http://careers.abpi.org.uk/working-in-the-industry/research/Pages/medical-writing.aspx. Accessed on October 18, 2017.

Sharma, S. How to become a competent medical writer? *Perspect Clin Res.* 2010;1(1): 33–37.

Whelan, J. *Medical Journalism – A Career Move?* The Write Stuff, The Journal of the European Medical Writers Association. http://www.emwa.org/documents/about_us/JA_V14_I2_Whelan1.pdf. Accessed on October 18, 2017.

PUBLIC SPEAKING

Jeroen van Baar

You are in front of a large audience. Warm stage lights flood your face and heat your torso. Why did you wear that jacket again? At least it helps to hide the sweat from your armpits. Your name is projected on the big screen. Everyone quietens down. The floor is yours.

Background

For a medical student today, this scenario is not uncommon. Public speaking is and will be an important part of your career, whether teaching, presenting scientific findings or speaking to a group of colleagues. Effective communication will be key even in your daily medical tasks and will be part of your research activities in the form of pitches for grants or presentations at interview. Yet public speaking is not formally taught in medical schools. That is why I was asked to write this chapter in the *Alternative Guide*. I am by no means a full-fledged *expert*, but I have gained relevant experience in writing and delivering speeches, pitching and chairing sessions; and as a cognitive neuroscience PhD student, I regularly give talks on 'the altruistic brain' to professional and lay audiences. I think public speaking is fun and useful, and I hope to share a strategy that will help you on your own public speaking journey: prepare, empathise and enjoy or 'PEE'. After a short description of this model, we will consider four common public speaking scenarios.

Prepare!

Proper preparation is invaluable for a successful public speaking experience. This may seem obvious, but that does not make it straightforward. It is easy to over-prepare for a long talk, which can render you rigid and unable to improvise to the audience's response. So how do you strike the right balance? In general, it is good to distinguish between preparing content and preparing delivery.

Content

For any talk over 5 minutes, you have to make sure that your story is worth listening to. Usually, this is bound to be the case: there is likely a good reason why you were invited to speak. So go back to basics. What is the main message that you want to confer to your audience? Which elements of information do they need in order to agree with you? And how can you structure these elements such that your argument runs smoothly and is enjoyable to listen to? You can never spend too much time on preparing content. If taking 30 minutes to add a video to your first slide improves your introduction – it is worthwhile doing.

Delivery

You can, however, spend too much time on preparing delivery. If you attempt to write down and memorise the exact phrasings and wordings of a speech, you are likely to lose focus once you make a single misstep. Suppose someone barges into the lecture hall or a light bulb drops from the ceiling 5 minutes after you have started – it is just awkward to ramble on with your well-prepared lines, pretending it did not happen. Preparing content, not delivery, will allow you to be flexible. The one exception to this rule is a situation in which your speech has very strict boundary conditions. At a TED conference, for example, most speakers have learnt their speech by heart because they have an exact time to fill and only get one shot at perfection. But even on TED, you sometimes see speakers stumble as they try to remember exactly which sentence was next. If possible, try to avoid this in everyday public speaking situations. Only actors and robots follow a script. Spend your time preparing content like the authentic speaker you are, and you will know how to express it when the time comes.

Empathise!

You are in front of that audience, and you have prepared your story perfectly. You know what you want to say. How do you make sure it hits home? The key here is empathy (and not just the emotional kind). When I was teaching physics to high school students as a side job, we learned to start each new topic by activating the class's prior knowledge. Talking about sound waves meant that we were building upon knowledge of not only energy, force and motion (physics), but also of sinuses (mathematics) and string instruments (music). By making these associations explicit, we helped the students embed what they were about to hear in their existing scaffoldings of memory. Your talk should do the same. You will teach your audience something new, but in order for them to understand it, you have to link it to what they already know. This also means that you should avoid jargon; and tailor your talk to the audience, otherwise you cannot expect others to follow you to your conclusion.

Top tip: Break the ice

One trick I have learned over the years is to chat a bit with the audience before you start your talk. This forms a bond with the crowd and gives you some social capital. If you have the time, introduce yourself in person to a few people in the front row. If you are in a panel, get acquainted with the other speakers. This will break the ice and help you be more comfortable on stage.

Enjoy!

We have all been to lectures that were interesting in content but simply lame to listen to. One sure-fire way to reach this result is by not enjoying yourself. Of course, this is easy for me to say – I find public speaking fun. But even if you dread being in front of an audience, the mindset you adopt can make all the difference. In a way, public speaking is comparable to waiting at the airport. Most people hate waiting for their flight, but there is a vast variation in the behaviour people exhibit at the gate. Some people retreat into their phones, some throw tantrums and some simply make the best of it by racing each other on the luggage carts. It is this kind of optimism that I am trying to get at. If you are into corny word puns, use them in your talk! If you are crazy about football, use examples from the World Cup in your speech! Even if your audience does not enjoy the puns or the examples, your genuine excitement will entice them to listen. Just as a speaker is supposed to empathise with the crowd, the crowd will empathise with an authentic speaker: if you enjoy yourself, others will too.

Anecdote: Shake things up

In 2014, I published a short book on achievement anxiety among young people in the Netherlands and the psychological consequences of it. One rainy evening later that year, I was at a high school in the city of Den Bosch to talk with parents about this topic. As I was giving my introductory lecture, something was off. I heard myself repeat the exact same phrases I had uttered some thirty times before, and nothing about my talk was inspiring anymore. My story had become boring to myself – and therefore to the audience. After this experience, I learned to prepare a new angle each time. Gearing my story to the audience and the occasion at hand makes it more interesting to listen to and much more fun to tell. So if you are giving the same talk multiple times, try to freshen it up periodically.

Four scenarios

Hopefully, the PEE model will be of use to you when you prepare or give a talk. But when will you do so? There are four scenarios that I want to outline.

Professional presentation

This is likely the most common format for a talk. Think of sharing research results at a conference, presenting a plan at a business meeting or giving a lecture at a high school or library. For this scenario, note that your entire argument is only as strong as its weakest component. If the audience does not buy the premise of your presentation, they are

Top tip: Show, do not just tell

An argument is most compelling if you give your audience the evidence that convinced you of it in the first place. For example, do not simply say that drug A alleviates symptom B – show a graph of the decline of symptom B. Do not state the gist – present the evidence. This strategy has a couple of important effects. Firstly, you show respect to the crowd, since you take them seriously. Secondly, your story will be much more entertaining if you let the audience draw their own conclusions. Lastly, you are putting yourself on the line, as a listener might draw a different conclusion from the evidence than you. This vulnerability, paradoxically, makes you strong and makes your story credible.

unlikely to believe the rest of it, and they might end up trying to think of clever objections instead of listening to what you have to say. In general, it is helpful to view these presentations as not too different from a sales pitch, the goal is the same: persuading or convincing your audience. Make sure the evidence with which you build up your argument is varied in nature. You can use everyday examples, anecdotes, quotes from experts, research findings, thought experiments, graphs, videos and so on. Finally, make sure you adhere to the formalities: keep good time; introduce yourself appropriately and thank the host; and at the end, acknowledge collaborators or funders and thank the audience. Leaving contact details or Twitter handles will mean people can get in touch with you afterwards.

Hosting/compering an event

Over the coming years, you might find yourself chairing a session at an academic conference or MC'ing at your best friend's wedding. Public speaking opportunities of this kind are really fun, because you get a lot of freedom. Of course, you will probably have to introduce the speakers or the bride's father, and you may have to chair question-and-answer (Q&A) sessions. But other than that, there are no guidelines on the style of MC'ing that you employ. Feel free to be yourself.

Focusing on academic or professional events, the foundation to doing well is to be – yes you guessed it – prepared. You have to know what the speakers are talking about if you are to steer the Q&A session in a meaningful direction. Good preparation will also help you think of appropriate questions in case no one in the audience has any and there is an awkward silence to fill. Aside from preparation, try to be of aid to the speakers: ask if they need any help setting up their presentation, if they want some water etc. This has a couple of neat effects: it will lower the expectation the audience has of your insight in the subject matter, as you are not held by the same standards as an expert; it will help you strike the right tone (naive and interested); and it will help combat nerves (usually the speaker I am helping is even more nervous than I am!). In general, it is important to dare to be vulnerable in your attitude at the event you are hosting. After all, your goal as a host is to make sure your guests get the most out of their attendance. By presenting yourself as naive and asking basic questions, you will create an open atmosphere in which participants feel comfortable asking the questions that will be most informative for them. Finally, by formulating several take-home messages at the end of the event, you can further promote this goal as the lights go down.

Delivering a pitch

Imagine you develop the next big innovation in diabetes treatment. How are you going to make sure that patients, investors and healthcare professionals take interest in your product? A good pitch is essential for reaching this goal. Here, you drive home one message in a matter of minutes. These restrictions have several important consequences for the way you go about your preparation. As a pitch is not always accompanied by slides, you want to ensure that your audience remembers you and your message well based on your words alone. Your pitch must be simple and strong. It is often helpful to start with a hook – personal rather than impersonal introductions are likely to cut through (see Box 4.4).

In a pitch, repetition will help you structure and ram home your message. As in every other public speaking scenario, your tone of voice must match its content. Finally, aim for the ending to be climatic: a firm call to action, another meeting with your audience or an invitation to invest in or purchase your product. If you do not ask, you will not get!

Giving a speech

A speech is the ultimate free-form public speaking opportunity. Like MC'ing, speeches are not bound to any particular context. And as with MC'ing, being yourself is the most important predictor of a successful speech. Whether delivering a birthday speech to a close friend or addressing allies in a political protest, a personal speech will help you illuminate and engage with any occasion you find important.

Aside from your being open and honest, structure is essential. Like writing a blog (covered elsewhere in this chapter), you will need to bring audiences along with you on your journey. A good way to do this

---

Box 4.4   Hook

Blunt: 'Diabetes kills X per year and causes a range of other organ problems which affects people's quality of life. My invention will help people to monitor their blood sugar digitally, which will reduce the number of people with poorly controlled diabetes.'

Sharp: 'Judith is an 85-year-old independent lady with diabetes, like many, she worries about her blood sugar levels; with our invention she will be able to monitor them with ease on her smartphone, allowing her instead to focus on the things that matter to her.'

Extreme: 'Imagine, for a moment, life with diabetes. You have to monitor and manage your blood sugar levels multiple times, every day of every year. Allow your levels to dip for just a minute, and you could be in grave danger. How much would you give to take this worry away?'

---

is to open your speech with a metaphor, allegory or intriguing question, to which the rest of your story relates. You can use the middle part of the speech to fan out into appropriate detail, as long as you converge on the theme of your introduction at the end. If you use this diamond structure, what you say will be easy to follow by your audience, and your speech will have a finished or 'resolved' feel. That said, even the most beautiful speech is worthless if it does not make a point. Make sure you have one and know how best to articulate it.

You may be required to prepare your speech word for word or in note form, depending on the occasion and your memory skills. A fully written speech is usually reserved for instances where exact wording is likely to be quoted or written about – policy announcements and so on will often take this form. In any case, make sure to road test your draft with friends or colleagues and ensure that it is of the correct length for your speaking speed (remember, everyone usually speaks slightly quicker on the day).

Anecdote: Speeches to get inspired

A good tip for improving your speeches is to watch experts at work. College commencement addresses from the United States are usually excellent examples; Steve Jobs's address to Stanford

University is world famous, but my personal favourite is the speech entitled 'This Is Water' by David Foster Wallace. Wallace delivered it at Kenyon College on 21 May 2005, and it is available in audio on YouTube or in extended, printed form from Little, Brown and Company. The speech works, in my opinion, because Wallace creates structure and wonder with an allegory that beautifully captures his point. See the 'Further reading' section for more information.

How to get gigs

While I hope this chapter has given you some food for thought on public speaking, there is no more effective way to develop your skills than doing it for real. The last topic of this chapter deals with this. How do you get invited to give talks?

You should start by exploring the public speaking landscape in your immediate environment. At every university, medical school and local library, there are a range of symposia each week. Attending these and offering to assist or chair sessions is a good first step towards giving talks more often. But if you want to be invited to speak publicly, you need to develop an expertise of your own. By writing a book, popularising what you have learned in medical school or capitalising on your personal experience, you can create a story that people want to hear and only you can tell.

Once you figure out what your unique angle is, you can start marketing yourself. There are many ways to go about getting your name out. For example, you can get registered at an agent for professional public speakers. Next to finding an agent, you can market yourself by contributing articles to newspapers and magazines, visiting conferences or being active on social media. You will be surprised how many event organizers are on Twitter!

Conclusion

To start public speaking, do not wait until you consider yourself an expert. Develop your skills early and in tandem with your wider profile. The more comfortable you become with a topic, the abler you are to speak on it to other people. As the editor for my own book often reminded me: expertise is not the starting point of a book, but rather the result. The same goes for public speaking. So good luck! And do not forget to PEE.

Common pitfalls

1. *Thinking nerves are bad.*

   Giving a talk to a professional audience is a nerve-wrecking activity for everyone. And that is totally OK so nobody expects you to be perfect out there. In fact, anxiety only makes your talk better! I rarely give a lecture without feeling nervous beforehand. Do not think that you can iron out your stress by over-preparing, either. For me, nerves usually follow proper preparation. Try to harness the energy and enjoy!

2. *Trying to keep ice-cold composure.*

   The only thing that matters is to convince your audience. Showing your nerves, breaking the ice and admitting that you are only human will help you reach that goal. If you have experience in science, you have probably attended one or two methodological talks where the speaker totally knew what they were doing and yet managed to deliver their story so arrogantly that no one felt like taking their advice to heart. In the end, public speaking is a social activity, and you will be successful if you manage to connect with the crowd.

3. *Starting your performance on stage.*

   A public speaking performance does not start when the first word is spoken, but much earlier. From the moment you enter the building where you are about to speak, the game is on. You might meet members of your audience in a hallway, or be introduced by a session chairperson when you are still sitting at the back of the room. Do not overthink it, but assume your role from the moment you set foot in the door.

4. *I am no genius.*

   If your presentation goes well, you may be asked a range of questions. At this point, it is yours to lose. You will often reach the point

Top tips: Ten steps to success in any presentation

1. Prepare content, not delivery.
2. Dress appropriately.
3. Get acquainted with the audience.
4. Be aware that your performance starts well before you take the stage.
5. Deliver with empathy and enjoyment.
6. Dare to improvise.
7. Thank the organisers.
8. Reflect on your performance.
9. Shake things up.
10. Repeat!

where you cannot answer a question from the audience. By simply saying you do not know, instead of frantically trying to formulate a reply that makes you seem smart, you simultaneously compliment the questioner on their curiosity and improve your own likeability and credibility by being honest.

Further reading (and inspiration)

American Rhetoric. https://www.americanrhetoric.com. [Online repository of famous speeches in the USA (PDFs and audio files).]

Barnett-Vanes, A., and De'Ath, H. *Presenting and Publishing as a PhD Student in 'How to Complete a PhD in the Medical and Clinical Sciences'*, 1st Edition. Wiley–Blackwell, Hoboken, NJ, 2017.

Clinton, H. Women's Rights are Human Rights (Speech). United Nations World Conference. 1995.

Hall, G., and Robinson, N. *How to Present at Meetings*, 3rd Edition. Wiley–Blackwell, Hoboken, NJ, 2011.

King, M. L. I Have a Dream (Speech). Washington, DC. 1963. [The speech makes unequalled use of pathos, pace, repetition, tone and metaphor. Note that much of his imagery stems from the Bible, which made sense in the Civil Rights Movement at the time. When applying metaphors in your own speeches, make sure that they sit well with the audience's look on life; otherwise, the most ornate idiom will be meaningless. In other words, empathise!]

TED. https://www.ted.com/. [A wealth of inspiring lectures from around the world.]

CHAPTER 5

Global health

CONTENTS

DEFINING AND MAPPING GLOBAL HEALTH

Azeem Majeed

Global health focusses on the increasing interconnectedness of health, including its wider determinants, across the world. In particular, recent decades have seen the rise of new global health challenges because of sweeping environmental, lifestyle and technological changes. For example, the rapidly rising global prevalence of obesity has led in turn to an increase in the prevalence of type 2 diabetes, which has imposed a considerable strain on societies, health systems and individuals. Meeting this global rise in non-communicable diseases and their risk factors is now a priority for international organisations such as the United Nations (UN) and the WHO, as well as for national governments.

Environmental changes such as global warming and drought have also resulted in new challenges for global health, such as the compromising of water supplies and increasing risk of diarrhoeal diseases. At the same time, the 'traditional' global health problems such as human immunodeficiency virus (HIV), malaria, other neglected tropical diseases and malnutrition still have a considerable mortality and morbidity burden, particularly in the countries of sub-Saharan Africa. Despite major improvements in health in recent decades, there remain large disparities in the health status between countries and by factors such as people's socio-economic status and educational level within countries. Addressing these health inequalities is another major challenge for organisations and individuals working to improve global health.

In today's very interconnected world, knowledge of the key global health challenges the world faces is important for medical students and training doctors. The increased levels of migration we have observed in recent decades have meant that many individuals from low- and middle-income countries are now living in higher-income countries. At the same time, the rapid development and reduced costs of air transport has resulted in increased levels of global tourism, thereby placing people from high-income countries at risk of acquiring diseases that were once rare among them. We also see the fragility of global health security – such as the recent Ebola epidemic and the rise of Zika disease – that requires a well-coordinated and multinational response to address effectively.

Hence, knowledge of the key principles of global health is now an essential component of undergraduate medical courses. This chapter provides a thorough grounding by highlighting opportunities and offering guidance on areas such as internships, research and medical electives in global health. Those with a special interest can continue their studies with postgraduate courses – as discussed elsewhere in this book – and clinical placements in low- and middle-income countries. As well as providing valuable knowledge and experience, such training also makes doctors well placed for a career in global health, either in research or in the many government, non-governmental and international organisations that work in this field (see Figure 5.1). Accordingly, we hope this chapter plays a role in expanding your global health horizons.

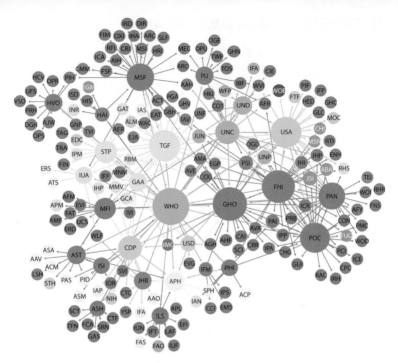

Node size is ranked by degree; node colour is partitioned by type of actor; and edges are coloured by source node.

- Global civil society organizations and NGOs
- Professional associations
- Public-private partnerships
- National governments
- UN system and intergovernmental
- Private industry
- Academic institutions
- Philanthropic organizations
- Multilateral development banks

Figure 5.1 Mapping global health institutions. (From Hoffman, S. J. et al., *Mapping Global Health Architecture to Inform the Future*, Chatham House, London, 2015.)

Acknowledgements

We are grateful to Chatham House, the Royal Institute of International Affairs, for the permission to reproduce Figure 5.1, originally published in the paper of Hoffman et al. [1].

Reference

1. Hoffman, S. J., Cole, C. B., and Pearcey, M. *Mapping Global Health Architecture to Inform the Future*. Chatham House, London, 2015.

INTERNSHIPS IN GLOBAL HEALTH

Vernon Lee and Moa Herrgård

Background

Undertaking internships in a global health institution is one of the most fascinating activities for medical students and health trainees. Global health institutions (Figure 5.1) provide a unique perspective on medicine that cannot be found in books, lectures or clinical rotations. As internships can range from 5 weeks to 6 months, you may not always be around for long enough to make substantial contributions to global health activities; however, there is still much you can both offer and learn from these opportunities.

Interning

Why?

An internship offers insight into the everyday life of a global health professional and, as such, is invaluable for anyone considering working in this field. They enable you to contribute to global health programmes and projects and provide you with the unique opportunity to network with healthcare workers and policymakers.

Where?

Internships include working in the field developing and strengthening local health systems and participating in clinical and epidemiological work or working at the headquarters on global health polices and engagements. Fieldwork provides insight to the problems facing lower-resource areas and exposure to issues such as health emergencies, infectious diseases surveillance and management, hygiene and sanitation. This includes building local capacities and providing community education with limited resources. Work at the headquarters provides perspectives on how these issues are collectively addressed by policy recommendations, collaborations across organisations and securing donor resources and funding.

UN agencies have country, regional and global offices. The majority of headquarters are located in New York (United States) and Geneva (Switzerland). Both cities are expensive to live in, and you may face challenges with visa requirements. It may be less competitive to receive an internship within a country or regional office; however, this may alter the type of work you can engage in. Alongside UN agencies and global health organisations, national or quasi-state

Table 5.1 High-profile global health agencies offering internships

Global health agency	Headquarters location (city, country)	Website
WHO	Geneva, Switzerland	http://www.who.int/employment/internship/en/
Global Fund to Fight AIDS, Tuberculosis and Malaria	Geneva, Switzerland	https://serviceinternships.com/internship/the-global-fund-internship-program/
Global Alliance for Vaccines and Immunization	Geneva, Switzerland	http://www.gavialliance.org/careers/internship-policy/
The United Nations Population Fund	New York, United States	http://web.unfpa.org/employment/internship.html
World Bank	Washington, DC, United States	http://www.ii.uam.es/intranet/WB Speech.pdf http://tinyurl.com/cfmfzd4
United Nations Programme on HIV/AIDS	Geneva, Switzerland	http://tinyurl.com/phq4qn3
United Nations Children's Fund	New York, United States	http://www.unicef.org/about/employ/index_internship.html
Global Health programme at the Bill & Melinda Gates Foundation	Seattle, United States	http://www.gatesfoundation.org/Jobs/Internship-Program-FAQ
United Nations Development Programme	New York, United States	http://www.undp.org/content/undp/en/home/operations/jobs/internships.html

Note: Details and websites are accurate as of 2016.

bodies also accept interns, including national health institutes, permanent missions and ministries of health. These opportunities may be more suitable for those seeking to forge a career within a specific country or region. Even if you do not pursue a career in global health, these skills are highly valued when working in local hospitals and health systems. Table 5.1 details some of the global health organisations offering internships.

Obtaining an internship

Theoretically an internship can be done at any time before, during or after your studies. Eligibility criteria vary depending on the institute, agency or organisation you are applying to. You will need to

Top tip

Do not be afraid to aim and apply for an internship in an institution which does not specifically work with just global health; the nexus approach of development and health is both attractive in the job market and broadens your experience.

demonstrate a level of technical knowledge in order to be able to conduct meaningful work duties; for this reason, you may find that many organisations require you to be a graduate student.

Yet, obtaining an internship is not as onerous as you may think. Yes, there are often many applicants (sometimes numbering into the thousands) to popular organisations, so the key is to present a CV that is different from the others. What are the unique attributes about yourself and how do you stand out from the crowd? Be specific about what you want to do and the experience you are looking for, and it will be easier for mentors to select you. Remember that mentors are looking for interns who are a good match in terms of interest and skills and can contribute to the team as much as they will learn from the experience. If you can find out the name and contact number of the mentor you would like to work for, direct contact is more personal and helps secure you a hearing. Networks are also important – if you know someone who works in the organisation (or someone who can link you with them), that would help in reaching out to the right mentor. See Box 5.1 for an application strategy.

Box 5.1   Shortlisting and application strategy

1. *Expectations*
   List the expectations you have for your internship, such as the following:
   a. Gaining insight into the work of a global health professional
   b. Contributing to improved global health provision now and in the future
   c. Improving your academic or technical knowledge
2. *Resources*
   List the resources you have at your disposal such as the following:
   a. Technical skills
   b. Knowledge and experience
   c. Connections and networks
   d. Direct and indirect financial resources

3. *Shortlist potential internships*

   Shortlist the institutions, agencies and organisations which interest you and narrow down on the specific departments within these. Where available, read the intern work descriptions or experiences of previous interns.

4. *Apply for the internship through formal and informal channels*

   Complete the online application for your target organisation(s) ensuring that you meet all necessary requirements. To maximise your chances of success, after making an official application, you may consider e-mailing the department or supervisor directly, informing them of your application and a short argument as to why you are interested and why they should select you. Remember to be modest but confident at the same time.

5. *Keep trying*

   If you do not receive a response – do not give up. It can take anywhere between a week to a year before you receive a response (if ever). This is because organisations are often inundated with applicants and fairly light on administrative personnel. That said, thousands of people intern in global health organisations each year, so keep trying. If you are unsuccessful, keep working to strengthen your skills and CV and prepare for another application.

Logistical and technical preparation

If you are successful in applying, congratulations! But the hard work has only just begun; you need to make sure you can get there first. Your first calling point will be to organise your accommodation, flights and visa – see Boxes 5.3 and 5.4 later in this section for an itinerary when going abroad. You may consider asking your supervisor or intern associations for online platforms to find accommodation. Be careful; interns are a common target for scammers – never transfer large sums of money in advance of arriving at your accommodation. See a list of associations at the end of this chapter for further resources. Many internships are currently unpaid and thus restrict access to many qualified candidates who cannot afford it [1]. As such, you will often need to secure your own funding. This may come from your savings, family or friends. However, most students find themselves raising their funds

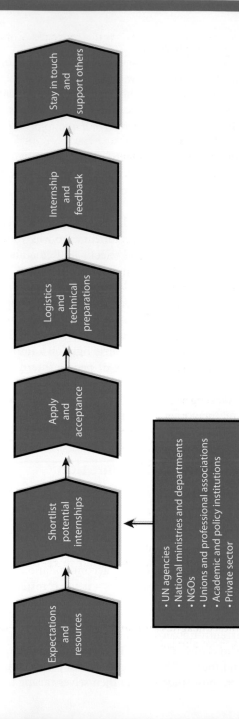

Figure 5.2   Internship lifecycle.

through a combination of scholarships, grants and loans. Contact your university well in advance for advice, including whether they can offer you support.

Finally, when taking up an internship position, it is likely that you will receive a terms of reference or TOR letter, detailing what duties you will have. Read up on your work duties and ask your supervisor to share suggestions for pre-reading materials. The more you know about the work carried out by the department ahead of starting the internship, the more you can offer once you arrive. Figure 5.2 summarises this application and logistical process.

Making a success of it

So what do you do once you are there? Being an intern means that you have substantial access to activities, meetings and projects, which will be an intriguing and educational experience. Do bear in mind that as much as your mentor would like to teach you all the ropes, he/she is also busy with many other tasks – you can build good will early on by assisting them. An internship is like a partnership, and everyone is looking for a win-win-situation. Ask your mentor what you can assist with, let him/her know about your interests so that you can be assigned relevant tasks and be enthusiastic about your work, even though it might seem mundane at first. Like all activities, you may need to start off doing and proving yourself at routine work before you can be assigned more complicated tasks. Do not be afraid to ask questions if you are unsure of anything and feel free to contribute your opinion – interns can provide invaluable perspectives and solutions to issues that staff may be unable to solve.

Finishing up and leaving

As you approach your final weeks, it is important that you prepare to leave. You may have arranged to meet or speak to certain colleagues or staff members during your internship – if any of these are outstanding, make sure you wrap them up. Offer to keep in touch with your colleagues, supervisors or mentors. In addition, ask your supervisor to provide you with feedback before the end of the internship, a certificate and a letter of recommendation. Maintain contact with your supervisor and colleagues and offer to meet them whenever you are in town. Keep them abreast too of any new publications or work outcomes.

Five top tips

1. *Achieve a balance of work duties.*
   Discuss with your supervisor your interests and ask to be given a range of tasks including ones that are both administrative and more substantive.
2. *Join an intern association.*
   These are a great source of academic, social and pastoral support. Many will be run by current or former interns and can offer you support on housing, intern work and life in the city.
3. *Never be afraid to ask for help.*
   As an intern, you are the most junior member of staff on the team. Never do anything you are unsure of or uncomfortable about without getting approval first. Pay attention to all organisational rules and regulations, especially on areas such as your institutional e-mail account.
4. *Apply only for internships you are interested in.*
   It can be tempting to tick as many boxes as possible when applying online, but you are not going to get much out of an internship whose work you do not care about. Focus your applications to those that you hold genuine interest in.
5. *What to do if you keep struggling to obtain an internship.*
   Alongside applying directly, there are many student organisations that facilitate access to internships. For example, the International Federation of Medical Student Associations offers members the chance to intern at WHO.

Outcomes

During the course of your internship, you may have contributed to academic work from your department which could lead to your inclusion as an author on papers, briefings or guidelines and so on. Alongside this, you will be in the position to write on your experience as an intern for a university newsletter, magazine or journal. This also offers you the chance to share and promote similar opportunities among peers and colleagues. For example, you can deliver short peer-to-peer workshops or give a presentation to other students.

Conclusion

Undertaking an internship in global health offers unrivalled insight into and experience working at the cutting edge. You get the chance to contribute meaningfully to global health work. If you are able to take up your internship, the opportunities available to you can be a platform to do a lot of good. Finally, do not forget to be part of the team and build your networks while you are there. Above all, enjoy yourself – it is all about learning and making a meaningful contribution.

Reference

1. Barnett-Vanes, A., Feng, C., Jamnejad, M., and Jun, J. Towards an equitable internship programme at WHO: Is reform nigh? *BMJ Global Health* 2016;1:e000088. doi:10.1136/bmjgh-2016-000088.

Further reading

Geneva Intern Association. http://internsassociation.org/.

Glocals. http://www.glocals.com/. For housing and living in Geneva.

International Federation of Medical Students Associations. http://ifmsa.org/.

UN Careers. Jobs and internships. https://careers.un.org/lbw/home.aspx ?viewtype=ip.

World Health Organization Intern Association. http://whointernboard.wixsite .com/whointerns.

GLOBAL HEALTH RESEARCH

Rose Penfold

Background

Global health research is defined as 'the area of study, research and practice that places a priority on improving health and achieving equity in health for all people worldwide' [1]. Howsoever it is defined, global health research aims not only to generate knowledge but also to initiate action. It raises public awareness of health issues in both developed and developing countries and is important in informing disease prevention and treatment strategies. High-quality research allows global agencies, governmental organisations, policymakers and NGOs to identify barriers to well-intentioned healthcare programmes and collect health metrics to measure the impact of interventions. Through research, sustainable and collaborative partnerships can be forged between health communities, supporting researchers in low- and middle-income countries in a way which is sustainable and self-reinforcing.

This chapter outlines some of the key considerations for any student wishing to undertake research in this rapidly expanding field. On a personal level, global health research facilitates opportunities to travel, to witness first-hand the delivery of healthcare in disparate settings and to interact with a network of scholars, journalists, healthcare professionals and medical educators around the globe. Bridging the healthcare gap requires collective action between as well as within countries; as a future member of the global medical profession, it is within your remit to contribute. But also take the time to evaluate your motives and ensure that your aims are realistic, feasible and address healthcare needs and deficits. Global health research is an exciting journey but a bumpy ride – so prepare yourself for a multitude of region-specific cultural, geopolitical and logistical barriers as well as many unanticipated hurdles along the way.

Logistical considerations
When?
Global health research can be conducted at any time, with focus appropriate for your current interests and stage of training. Decide whether your project is limited or ongoing, set clear targets and ensure that these are realistic and flexible. Do not underestimate the time it will take to liaise with organisations in other parts of the world, apply for travel grants and funding and obtain ethical approval. If your research involves on-the-ground work or data collection, you will need to factor in an additional period to travel, acclimatise and access necessary resources at the study site. Ensure that *your* team is able to complete the project. From experience, relying on healthcare professionals, future groups of elective students or others working in the region to finish data collection risks undermining all the hard work you have already done.

How to find and organise a project
The important message here is to be proactive: respond to adverts, look for relevant talks and presentations and speak to those experienced in the field. An easily accessible source of information is your fellow students and colleagues who have previously conducted research during electives, student-selected projects or vacations. Ask them how they organised their project, any problems encountered and their plans for future work. Many universities have a dedicated centre of research and teaching, such as a global health institute, which may already be running a range of projects with experience or networks in a given region. Alternatively, look at student groups and societies (for example, Students for Global Health or sections of the Royal Society of

Medicine in the United Kingdom). At the very least, they will provide a strong network of like-minded individuals who may expose you to new ideas, opportunities and sources of funding for your project.

Depending on the nature of your intended research, the traditional supervisor–student model may be less applicable here than in other fields of research. Having said this, setting up a successful project alone from scratch is challenging and ill-advised. By all means, do some background reading to identify areas of personal interest, in which you perceive research to be lacking. But consider the practicalities and seek advice from those with expertise in the area in which you wish to work. Aim to meet with several researchers to discover more about the work they are doing before embarking on a project; avoid taking on multiple new endeavours simultaneously or helping to data analyse/audit/write up without clear evidence that you will be adequately acknowledged. Do not be afraid to turn down projects which you perceive to be uninteresting or unrealistic or where your contribution will be undervalued. While the best supervisors are not necessarily the most senior, also be wary of relative newcomers to the field with much enthusiasm and novel ideas but a series of unsuccessful applications and incomplete projects to date. Have a look online or through PubMed at previous works or publications and who contributed to these to get some idea of what you might be taking on.

Ethical considerations

In addition to the usual considerations, be aware of the international controversy which surrounds ethics in global health research and the complex interplay between large-scale research collaborations in high-income countries and the ways in which research is conducted and manifested locally. External sponsors differ in their motives for research, and inequalities in resources between developed and developing countries pose potential risks of exploitation. Ensure that you adhere to local requirements. Most ethics committees now operate a principle of avoiding duplication (i.e. they accept ethics approval awarded by another committee), but this may not apply to approval from another country, where there is more limited information about the scrutiny process. Be aware of specific cultural, legal or social considerations in the region. For example, in some regions, it is expected that you seek permission from the community or an elder before approaching individuals for their individual consent, particularly women and children (but note that this should never override individual consent given by a competent adult). Before starting, it is worth reviewing the principles and recommendations of several policy-advising organisations such as WHO, Wellcome Trust and Nuffield Council of Bioethics Working Party.

Funding your research

A deterrent for many students contemplating global health research is the financial cost. Potential sources of funding depend on the focus and timing of your project, and it is not possible to produce an exhaustive list herein. If you are conducting research during a medical elective, student-selected project or an intercalated degree, university/ institution-specific bursaries may provide financial support. Also look for more widely available bursaries and prizes; each has different application criteria, often requiring specific project work and/or an extensive report to be written on your return. Think broadly about your chosen project – for example, does it have relevance for global mental health, primary care or women's health? Search online – do your research aims fall under the remit of any charities, research collaborations or academic institutions? There is no limit to the number of applications you can make, and the hours spent researching and drafting applications are often a fruitful time investment.

Furthermore, medical schools and funding bodies may offer monetary prizes to noteworthy projects. For those willing to put in the extra mile, prize essays and commentaries on your experiences may also be financially rewarded. Of course, you cannot rely on this funding when budgeting in advance, but any such money could be put towards essential resources for continuation of the project. That said, apply for these strategically and avoid a scattergun approach; note that deadlines will often fall a long way in advance of your intended research period. Furthermore, you do not want the scope and deadlines of your project to be constrained by the need to meet strict funding body requirements. Carefully select a few sources of funding and target your applications accordingly.

A final point to mention here is that not all international research needs to be costly. The emergence of innovative web-based solutions for global communication and their expansion in developing countries is making long-distance partnership and remote research or intervention increasingly feasible.

Anecdote: Utilising innovative web-based technology

OxPal is a distance-learning partnership between students and faculty in Oxford, United Kingdom, and the occupied Palestinian territories. The OxPal research group conducted fieldwork to assess the learning needs of the students and the unique geopolitical barriers to medical education and to evaluate initial pilot tutorials of the programme. Real-time tutorials are delivered via an innovative online platform featuring smartboard, audio/video and instant messenger. Evaluation via online questionnaires has consistently demonstrated tutorials to be useful and locally relevant.

OxPal demonstrates that global research and intervention can be feasibly conducted remotely and at a low cost.

Completing your research

It is inappropriate and unhelpful to translate research findings directly from a more developed healthcare system to another with less funding and resources. When formulating your project, do some background research. What *general* and *specific* barriers might you encounter? Geopolitical, cultural and language factors will all be relevant here. Background reading and talking to those who have worked in the region will give you a good understanding, but there is no substitute for spending time there yourself to appreciate first-hand the specific healthcare needs and problems you might encounter. To give a few examples, think about the timing of your research – do not expect rapid responses to e-mails during the holy month of Ramadan in countries where this is a national holiday. Poor public transport links may mean you have to limit research to a single rather than multiple sites. A lack of basic supplies may necessitate your project temporarily grinding to a halt while a hospital tackles a supply issue. You may face hostility from native healthcare workers and struggle to recruit locals if you do not adequately convey the purpose and potential benefits of your research. Depending on where you are working, it may take time to adapt to the heat or the climate; despite meticulous preparation, you may still succumb to a travelling-related illness. Furthermore, be prepared that the difficulties you predict may not be the same as those you encounter – demonstrated in the following anecdotal account.

**Anecdote: Can an early warning score be used
to predict 24-hour mortality in a regional hospital
in Malawi?**

The UK National Early Warning Score (EWS) provides a surveillance system for monitoring the condition of in-patients. A group of elective students looked at introducing this score in a regional hospital in Malawi, one of the world's poorest countries. A focus group with local healthcare professionals outlined score calculation and what further actions may be indicated. Next day, on the ward, EWS was inaccurately calculated. Why? The wards lacked basic observation equipment and printing paper; nurses were not adequately trained. Having modified the score and demonstrating that it does predict mortality, the task was then to initiate change by working with local healthcare professionals in the region.

Lesson: Perform background research and check the suitability of your project on the ground in advance.

Disseminating your research

Finally, after weeks, months or years, you are in a position to showcase your work. How do you disseminate your findings to a wider audience and suggest interventions to bring about change? Think about your target population and the messages you wish to send; look for conferences and journals which have accepted similar work previously. Think broadly and realistically, considering regional, national and international forums. Involve your co-workers in the writing-up process and ensure those that do not merit authorship – but were important nonetheless – are acknowledged.

Journals

It may be unrealistic to aim straight for *Lancet Global Health* or *Journal of Epidemiology and Global Health*. Instead, perhaps consider journals with a more specific focus for your region or research topic. Aim to emulate the style of the journal when writing, but be prepared to extensively redraft or resubmit elsewhere if your work is not accepted.

With an ever-changing and increasingly diverse range of journals publishing original research, reviews, commentaries, project reports and blogs relating to aspects of global health, it is unhelpful and unrealistic to list all here. Table 5.2 presents just some of the journals referenced

Table 5.2 Popular global health journals

Journal	Focus
Journal of Epidemiology and Global Health (JEGH)	Special interest in global health policies, where these have been implemented based on epidemiological and public health research. Focus on priorities of the World Health Assembly. JEGH will not accept case reports or pure basic (bench) science reports.
The Lancet Global Health	Original research, commentary, correspondence, blogs on topics including reproductive, maternal, child health, infectious and neglected tropical diseases, mental health, global health workforce and systems and policy in low-/middle-income countries. High impact factor.
Medicine, Conflict and Survival	Medical and psychological issues related to conflict, violence and human rights.
Journal of Global Health	Original research and review articles, personal viewpoints, research protocols, editorials and news in two issues per year. Edinburgh University Global Health Society.
Pan-African Medical Journal	Original research, reviews, commentary on current health initiatives; project reports; and personal experiences commenting on clinical, social, political, economical factors affecting health in Africa. Online, rapid and free availability.
Journal of Public Health in Africa	High-quality original articles and reviews on public health-related issues in Africa.
Medical Teacher	Journal of AMEE, an international association for education in medical and healthcare professions. Accounts of new teaching methods, guidance on structuring courses and assessing achievement and forum for education-related communication.
Global Health, Science and Practice	Focusses on lessons learned and the *how* of global health programmes, aiming to improve health practice especially in low-/middle-income countries.
Central Asian Journal of Global Health	Online open access journal; discussion of public health; and medicine and global health reviews, perspectives and news, particularly in Central Asia. Supportive environment for new investigators and those who have never published in English language journals.
International Journal of MCH and AIDS	Research and review articles, clinical and evaluation studies, policy analyses, commentaries and opinions in maternal, infant, child health and HIV/AIDS in low-/middle-income countries and those with health disparities. Focus on social determinants of health and disease.

(Continued)

Table 5.2 (Continued)   Popular global health journals

Journal	Focus
Annals of Tropical Paediatrics: International Child Health	Interest in child health in the tropics and subtropics, covering the whole range of diseases in childhood and the social, cultural and geographical background in which they appear. Aimed primarily at specialists in tropical medicine and infectious diseases, parasitologists and paediatricians.
BMJ Global Health	A recent addition to the global health journal family, accepts research, analysis, commentaries and letters on topics and research concerning global health.

Note: Details accurate as of 2017.

in the PubMed database, with their areas of focus. Remember to also look at the timescale and medium for publication and fees associated with each.

Presentations

Draft an abstract to submit to relevant regional and national conferences. Examples include the Unite for Sight Global Health and Innovation conference, the International Health Congress, the World Health Summit and the annual Consortium of Universities for Global Health (CUGH) conference. Universities, institutions and organisations such as the Royal Society of Medicine in the United Kingdom or CUGH in the United States also run specific global health events with abstract and essay submissions. Such forums are not only useful from a portfolio perspective but also provide the chance to network with others who share your passion for global health.

Driving change

However, while presentations, publications and prizes are vital for future job applications and career progression, do not lose sight of your overarching goal – to initiate change for improvement. Work with healthcare workers and the local population to educate and make changes to current practice. For example, you could present your findings to the hospital directorate or even to higher policymakers, NGOs and governmental organisations. Leave a legacy of sustainable and self-reinforcing impact while fostering relationships which you can build on in the future.

Post-research: What next?

Now you have collected and analysed your data, written up and published your findings, your work does not stop here. Make sure you follow up to see whether changes in policy or practice were implemented and, if so, the effect these have had. This is much easier in the current age of technology – collect e-mail addresses and details of local contacts before you leave. It is courteous and good practice to send any presentations or publications to all those involved, including local colleagues and policymakers with whom you collaborated. Remember, fostering international partnerships may aid future collaboration should you or others wish to continue research in the area.

Conclusion

There are myriad potential career benefits to global health research. With the opportunity to acquire transferable research skills, attend and present at national and international forums and build a worldwide professional network, it is no wonder that global health research is snowballing in popularity. Most importantly, however, global health research provides the opportunity to make a tangible impact to the lived experience and health conditions of people throughout the world. Although no amount of words can do justice to the rich and diverse personal experiences that lie in wait, I hope this chapter will be helpful as you embark on your own research journey in this challenging and dynamic field.

Common pitfalls

1. *Conflicting interests and research aims from organisations and funding bodies.*

   Be wary of involving too many third parties simultaneously.

2. *Violation of social and cultural expectations in region of work.*

   Do background research and spend time in communities where you are working.

Top tips

1. First and foremost, evaluate your motives and utility of your project. The overarching aim is to generate sustainable and self-reinforcing change.
2. Set realistic time frames, then add in further contingency time.
3. Make a list of potential political, cultural, social and ethical barriers and be prepared for unanticipated setbacks.
4. Foster long-term collaboration.
5. Involve local healthcare workers and present your findings locally.

3. *Translating research directly from developed to developing settings.*
   This inevitably will not address the most pressing healthcare needs.

4. *Failure to write up and disseminate findings appropriately – both to the local community and through presentation and publication.*

Further reading

Benatar, S., and Brock, G. (eds). *Global Health and Global Health Ethics.* Cambridge University Press, New York. 2011.

Cash, R., Wikler, D., and Saxena, A. (eds). *Casebook on Ethical Issues in International Health Research.* World Health Organization, Geneva. 2009.

Koplan, J. P. et al. Consortium of Universities for Global Health Executive Board. Towards a common definition of global health. *Lancet.* 2009; 373(9679):1993–5.

Opio, M. O. et al. Validation of the VitalPAC EWS Score (ViEWS) in acutely ill medical patients attending a resource-poor hospital in sub-Saharan Africa. *Resuscitation.* 2013;84(6):743–6.

Penfold, R. S. et al. Evaluation of the first year of the Oxpal Medlink: A web-based partnership designed to address specific challenges facing medical education in the occupied Palestinian territories. *JRSM Open.* 2014;5(2):2042533313517692. doi: 10.1177/2042533313517692.

The Global Health Book. Global Health: Investing in Our Future. InterAction: A United Voice for Global Change, 113th Congress. 2013. http://www.global health.org/wp-content/uploads/GlobalHealthBriefingBook_FINAL_web .pdf.

ELECTIVES: PLANNING

Katie Dallison

Background

You have just about finished medical school, and now, before you enter the challenging world of work, you may have the opportunity to go on an elective.* Your elective can help shape the rest of your

---

* The *elective* refers to a 6- to 10-week student clinical or research placement, usually conducted overseas in a medical student's final year. Depending on which country you are from, the name may differ.

career, providing a great base for future placements, training and job opportunities, and not to forget, the people you meet could go on to be lifelong friends. Realistically, this is one of the few opportunities in your career where you will have complete freedom of choice, to go where you want and meet whom you choose, so use it wisely! You will generally need to begin planning your elective at least 12 months in advance. I say at least, as think of all the other things that will happen in your final year – exams, practicals, placements. The list is endless, so the sooner you start, the better.

Where do I go for my medical elective?

This is the most common question I am asked by medical students in their penultimate year. The straightforward answer is wherever you like – you can literally go anywhere in the entire world! A far better first question to ask yourself is what do I want to learn from my elective? If you were applying for your first job as a doctor, what would you like to tell your future employer about your elective experience? Firstly, set yourself some good objectives. This will help your research and gives you a focus to return to when you start learning exciting things about exotic opportunities. If you plan to apply for funding, it also tells funding bodies that you are a serious candidate who has considered their options. See Box 5.2 for a few questions I think are important to answer; hopefully, they will help you to formulate three to four specific goals.

Anecdote: Your elective goals

One student I worked with decided her goals would be (1) to build three new network contacts within public health, (2) to better understand a different community and (3) to get a poster presentation. She could have gone to many places around the world to achieve this; however, after doing her research, she decided her best option was to work with a homeless charity based within 20 miles of her university. She achieved all her objectives, had a great time and has since used the contacts she made to arrange placements in other national and international homeless communities. Focusing on her objectives during her planning also helped her ask relevant questions of potential elective supervisors which no doubt highlighted to them how organised and mature she was about her elective.

Box 5.2   Ten big questions

1. Do I know what specialty I would like to go into? If so, how can I use my elective to build my portfolio towards this specialty? If not, how can I use my elective to explore different options?
2. Is there a particular area of research I am interested in?
3. Do I want to explore a different medical system? If so, why? And what do I want to know about it?
4. Do I want to build my network? If so, who or what area in particular?
5. Do I want to learn more about a specific medical technique?
6. Do I need to speak my patient's/team's language to enable me to interact with them? Or would I like the challenge of learning different communication skills?
7. What sort of immediate environment would I learn more from? Small clinic vs. large hospital? Many resources vs. few resources?
8. Is there a geographical region/country that I am considering working in in the future? How could I best use my elective to understand this more?
9. What else (non-clinical) do I want to achieve out of my elective?
10. Do I want to get anything specifically out of my elective, e.g. a poster presentation or the start of a paper?

What do I need to know?

Once you have set your objectives, you can begin your research into the huge range of opportunities available to you. At this early stage, I would suggest not getting too hung up on the very specific planning details – it is good to keep an open mind and identify a few different options to take through to the reality checking stage. Use your objectives to guide this research, always coming back to that central question of 'Will this get me what I want?' Generally, a good starting point is your university. Most universities will have a staff member (or a team) to help and guide your elective planning. If you are not told who this is, find out at least 12 months before you need to go on your elective as there should be a specific process to follow. In terms of beginning your research, universities usually have past elective reports that you can access, and they may even have their own database of potential contacts or opportunities. Using your university alumni network could allow you to contact someone who has done a similar elective in previous years which will give you invaluable first-hand knowledge (and another doctor to add to your ever-growing network).

The obvious place to research is on the internet. Always be aware of who has written the articles that you are reading. Are they trying to market an opportunity to you or is their information based on hard facts (complete with references)? If the article is from a personal account, do they mention any bad things or challenges they faced? If they do not, then be wary as there will always be challenges in new situations. Make some of your basic research about the medical systems in a country you are interested in, as this will help you to better define your searches to locate hospitals and clinics that fit with your elective objectives. Do not forget to keep checking in with your objectives to keep your research focussed.

Making use of your network is the best way to either learn about new opportunities, see opportunities from different angles or help you confirm your findings. Speak to anyone you know who has done an elective, especially when you are on clinical placements with junior doctors, as they will have information which will be current and thus most useful for you. Do not be afraid to contact people through social media, e.g. LinkedIn or via international or country-based networking communities like the International Medical Student's Federation, Medsin-UK or the American Medical Students Association.

And when it comes to making that initial contact with your potential elective supervisor, find out how they would like to be approached first. A quick phone call to their secretary or reception staff should help you with this. Once you have established contact, build your creditability by doing some research into their professional background. Use this research to ask some good questions about their work. This will show them that you have really put some time and thought into working with them and helps you establish if the elective will meet your objectives.

Reality checking

This is where it all starts to get real. You have your objectives, and through your research, you have identified a few different opportunities. Now it comes down to making this elective happen.

Visa

If you are planning to go overseas, there is no point in going to all the trouble of organising your perfect elective if you cannot get into the country. Part of your initial research will be to see if you can gain an entry visa. This depends on your own nationality and the country you wish to do your elective in. Visa rules can change, so check the embassy website of the country you intend to travel to. There are companies that can help you apply for visas (particularly if time is short), but often they are expensive, so use with caution. Be sure to include any visa costs in your budgeting (see Box 5.3).

Funding

Funding your elective is one of the main areas of concern for many medical students – see Box 5.3 for a breakdown of the costs involved. However, do not let the cost of your perfect elective put you off – there are quite a few funding opportunities out there. Further, the act of writing a funding bid (and winning that funding) looks great to future employers. The first thing you will have to do is write a budget so you know how much money you are going to need. The next task is to find funding opportunities. Try your university first – they often have ring-fenced funds available which will have less competition as it is only open to students from your specific university. You will generally want to apply for more than one grant or bursary (although check the rules and regulations of the funding provider, as sometimes this is not allowed). Explore medically related charities or websites specific to electives in your country. For example, in the United Kingdom, Money for Med Students (http://www.money4medstudents.org/) is run by the Royal Medical Benevolent Fund. Medical associations across the world can also highlight good funding opportunities. Check the requirements of the grant or bursary you are going to apply for and make sure you meet every requirement. Generally, you will need to prove you are a capable medical student (usually via a reference from an academic at your university and your CV) and that you have planned your elective down to the last detail. Get someone to double check your application before you submit it and make sure to add the date you can expect to hear back from them to your calendar. Sometimes this date can be very close to when you will need to confirm with your elective provider that you are going to arrive, so it is worth having a second option elective on the backburner to make sure you do not miss out.

Admin

With any situation where you come into contact with patients, there will be some form of clearance that you will be required to get before you can begin. For example, most hospitals will require you to attend an occupational health check, which many of you may have already experienced during your university placements. If you are travelling internationally, this step becomes even more important and could possibly prevent your travel or cause the cancellation of your elective. Read everything that you are sent regarding vaccinations, documentation and health checks you need to have before you leave. In terms of vaccines required by each country, you can find a comprehensive list here at Fitfortravel (http://www.fitfortravel.nhs.uk/) and double check with your university to see if they have any extra advice for you.

Box 5.3   Money, money, money

- Travel (flights, airport taxis, public transport)
- Visas
- Vaccinations/health checks before you go (and potentially, malaria tablets while you are there)
- Accommodation
- Food and drinks
- Indemnity insurance (if you need it – check details with the country you are travelling to and see if your medical school can help here)
- Travel insurance
- Basic first aid kit (and potentially, extra supplies if you are travelling to a resource-poor country)
- Any extra fees (if you are organising your elective through a company)
- Personal spending money (be sure to take into account currency exchange rates)

Finally, ensure that you have the following essentials in Box 5.4 ticked off in advance of your departure and see Table 5.3 for what to and not to do.

Box 5.4   Essential checklist

- *Documentation:* Passport; visa; insurance (both travel and indemnity); travel tickets; vaccination/health check certificates; verification that you are a university student (a letter from your university is usually the best option); addresses and contacts of where you are staying, your supervisor, and emergency contacts such as embassy details; international driver's licence (if required – check with the country you are traveling to); any other local paperwork you may need.
- *While you are on your elective:* Accommodation; a basic first aid kit (do not forget your stethoscope; torch; and medication such as anti-diarrhoea tablets, water purifying pills, rehydration products etc.); credit cards/local currency; electrical devices adapter plugs, power packs or spare batteries; medical books or reference guides you might need; personal items that might be hard to get hold of (e.g. personal medication, feminine hygiene products, your favourite chocolate bar); gifts you may like to give your elective team.

Table 5.3 Dos and don'ts: planning

Dos	Don'ts
Do start planning as early as you can – it will always take longer than you think!	Do not leave home without taking copies/photographs of all your documentation so you can always access them if needed.
Do set objectives and revisit them throughout your planning stages (as well as when you are on your elective).	Do not rely solely on online contact – if possible, arrange to phone or Skype your supervisor in advance. It is far more personal and makes your arrival more real both for yourself and them.
Do have a backup plan if relying on funding applications.	Do not forget to explore what other opportunities you might have for networking on your elective – experiences outside of your immediate department/unit are hugely valuable.
Do read everything that you are sent regarding your elective at least three times so you do not miss any important information.	

Further reading

http://www.wdoms.org/ [The world directory of medical schools – useful if you are interested in a research focused elective.]

http://www.who.int/hrh/resources/en/ [A range of resources developed by the WHO including statistics and information on many healthcare systems around the world.]

Medilexicon. http://www.medilexicon.com/medicalassociations.php [Listings of over 1200 medical associations and societies – useful as a starting point as most associations have guidance on electives, e.g. the British Medical Association (https://www.bma.org.uk/medicalelective).]

The Commonwealth Fund. http://www.commonwealthfund.org/ [Reports, statistics and research into various topics within international healthcare. Great place for inspiration.]

ELECTIVES: DOING

Tim Robinson

Background

After months of planning and countless e-mails, not to mention all those hours studying for exams, you have finally arrived at your destination ready to start your elective. This is the culmination of years at medical school, and for many people, a highlight of their time at university. Each person will have different objectives specific to their interests and potential career plan, and no doubt, the time you have spent planning your elective up to this point will go some way towards meeting these goals. However, there is only so much you can do before you arrive; now is the time to get stuck in and make sure you get the most out of your elective.

When you arrive

Hopefully, you will have arranged to meet someone at the airport who will take you to your final destination or, for the more intrepid among you, managed to find your way alone. If you are doing your elective abroad, particularly in a developing country, it will take a few days to acclimatise to the new environment. You will need to give yourself time to adjust to the time difference, move in to your accommodation, change any currency if you have not already done so and familiarise yourself with the local area.

You should already know your objectives and have a timeline of how you will go about achieving them, as discussed in the previous chapter. Try to meet your local supervisor in the first few days. This will give you a chance to discuss your plans in detail and go through the practicalities of your elective. Find out where you will be working and what is expected of you and try to meet the people you will be working with. If you can, have a look round the hospital/clinic before you start working there. The sooner you do all these things, the easier it will be when you start your placement or project.

Getting started

You will be working with new people in an unfamiliar setting, so it will take time to get to know your role. Do not expect too much initially. You should aim to observe as much as possible so that you get an idea of the normal practices and routines at the hospital/clinic and become acquainted with the customs of the local population (which might be very different to those you are used to and, as such, have a pronounced effect on health beliefs and behaviours). By the end of the first week, you should have started to get to know your colleagues and the way they work and feel comfortable in your new environment. In addition, you should have noted areas where you think you may be of benefit. Do not be alarmed if, despite all your planning, things do not turn out quite as you expected. No amount of preparation is a substitute for being there in person. Use the first week to try to identify any potential problems you had not anticipated. Be adaptable – we often learn far more when things go wrong than when everything runs smoothly.

Subsequent weeks

Now that you have established your role and got to know your colleagues, you should aim to go about achieving what you set out to do on your elective. If you are conducting research, you should be in a position to start collecting data; if your elective is based in a clinical environment, you should aim to gain as much experience as possible, be it observing or playing an active part in the healthcare team. The latter is especially true for those going to developing countries. One of the many reasons students choose to go to these areas is to gain hands-on practical experience. Much of the clinical knowledge we gain at medical school is through passive rather than active learning, and when I was a student, I often felt frustrated that I could not contribute more to the team. An elective offers a fantastic opportunity to put all the things you have learnt into practice. Try to make the most of everything you encounter and try to learn from the cases you come across.

You should aim to maintain regular contact with your home supervisor. Use them to troubleshoot any problems you encounter. They will be able to offer advice and, as your elective progresses, can help ensure that you are on target to achieve what you set out to do. Reflect on cases as you go and write down any memorable experiences so you do not forget them. Think about what you learnt and how you can apply this in the future.

Key considerations
Safety
The vast majority of people's electives run smoothly. Good planning is key, although even the best-prepared student may have the odd mishap. It may be stating the obvious, but be vigilant about personal safety and use common sense. Try to ensure that you travel with others, especially in the early stages of your elective when you may not be so familiar with your surroundings. If you do go anywhere alone, particularly for a long period, make sure you tell people where you are going and when you expect to be back. It is worth acquainting yourself with the local consulate or embassy and considering what you would need to do if, for whatever reason, you had to return home in an emergency.

Ethical dilemmas
There may be times when you are faced with difficult moral and/or ethical scenarios. For perhaps understandable reasons, such dilemmas tend to occur more frequently in resource-poor settings. Some students may have to confront the tricky prospect of being the most qualified person at the scene, with the knowledge that an adverse outcome may occur unless they intervene. Keep in mind the key principle of a physician: to do no harm. Ask yourself, 'Would I be doing this if I was in my home country?' If the answer is no, then you should not do it on your elective either. And while you should try to maximise your learning opportunities in the elective, this should never be to the detriment of the patients. If you feel that you are being asked to do things above your level of experience or expertise, say so. Do not be afraid to refuse

requests that you are not comfortable with. If you have any doubts, speak to your supervisor.

Finishing up

As the end of your elective approaches, hopefully, you will be in a position to look back on what you have achieved over the last few weeks. Whatever your personal and professional goals at the start, you should find that you have learnt a huge amount without even realising it. The theoretical and practical knowledge you have picked up, the patients you have seen and any unexpected challenges you have encountered along the way will no doubt stand you in good stead and leave you better prepared for life as a newly qualified doctor and beyond. Remember that you should not be the only beneficiary. Think about what you can do to ensure that some form of sustainability comes out of your elective. If you have done research, make sure you disseminate the findings to your colleagues. If you have set up a new project or initiative, is there someone who will be able to continue it after you leave? Speak to other students at your medical school so that they can use your contacts in the future. Stay in touch with your hosts after you leave – you never know what opportunities may arise later in your career, and it pays to have a network of people across various parts of the globe.

Most medical schools require you to write a report when you get back from your elective. This may seem like a chore, but it should not be too taxing and actually represents a great opportunity to aim for a publication. If you did research, have a look at the relevant journals related to your subject area (see Table 5.2). Your supervisor should be able to help with this. There is also a scope for publication of reflective pieces – you just need to look in the right places [1]. When writing your report, you should find the notes you made at the time useful to jog your memory; alternatively, the e-mails you sent to your family and/or supervisor should act as a good reminder of events.

Conclusion

Your elective is a unique chance to broaden your horizons in a different and perhaps unfamiliar environment, gain new skills and develop specific areas of interest. See Table 5.4 for key dos and don'ts. Enjoy it and use it wisely – it may shape the rest of your career.

Table 5.4 Dos and don'ts on elective: doing

Dos	Dont's
Push yourself and take advantage of the learning opportunities you encounter.	Do not expect too much too soon – give yourself time to get to know people and become familiar with the environment.
Keep focussed on your objectives and make sure that you are on track to meet them.	Do not do anything you do not feel comfortable doing – if you have any doubts, tell someone.
Stay in touch with people at home – family, friends and your supervisor.	Do not be put off by setbacks – these are just as useful as anything you planned.
Make the most of your free time to travel and explore the country.	Do not forget that local customs may be very different to the ones you are familiar with back at home.

Reference

1. Robinson, T. Lessons from an elective in Sierra Leone. *Pan African Med J.* 2014;17:181. [This is a reflective article I wrote and published after my elective.]

Further reading

Studentbmj. http://www.student.bmj.com/student/section/careers/electives.html.

The Electives Network. Case studies. https://www.electives.net/cases.

ELECTIVES: PERSPECTIVES

Harvard Medical School Exchange Clerkship Program

Saori Koshino

My academic objective in applying to the Exchange Clerkship Program of Harvard Medical School (HMS) was to obtain knowledge of neurology and radiology in the high-yield setting. I had already developed a track record in imaging studies: winning first prize in the Japan Science & Engineering Challenge, representing Japan at the Intel International Science & Engineering Fair and publishing my functional magnetic

Top tips

- Think globally, act locally.
- Be a self-starter.
- When you hear hoofbeats, think horses, not zebras.
- Take it easy!
- Be ambitious!

resonance imaging neuro-imaging research in a peer-reviewed medical journal following my BSc research project at Imperial College London. These experiences strengthened my candidacy for the Exchange Clerkship Program.

My medical school, Tokyo Medical and Dental University, assisted in organising the application and offered training in history taking, physical examination, oral presentation and critical thinking. They also supported me in the telephone interview preparation and English Language examinations. I was successful at the interview and rotated through advanced study in neurology at Beth Israel Deaconess Medical Center and paediatric radiology at Boston Children's Hospital.

Thanks to the convenient accommodation and location, it was not too difficult to adjust to this environment, even though the morning ward round started at 7 a.m.! During the neurology rotation, I saw patients with a range of neurological conditions; my work included history taking, physical examination, progress note writing, oral presentation and consultation with other departments. On radiology, I saw a range of cases and, at my request, spent 3 weeks at the neuroradiology department. Alongside clinical work, I also attended an educational conference held every day with HMS students and participated in student presentations and meetings.

My ambition is to become a world-leading neuroradiologist, and my elective at HMS has undoubtedly contributed towards this aim. My advice is simple: if you see an opportunity, take it!

University of Oxford Medical School Elective

Osaid H. Alser

As a fourth-year medical student from Gaza in Palestine, I decided to visit a highly developed country with a state-of-the-art medical training system to undertake my elective clinical training. For me, there was no better place to do this than at Oxford University – seen by many as the best in the world. Electives in the United Kingdom enable visiting medical students from across the world to visit its universities and experience first-hand the NHS. I duly completed the application process online and, to my delight, received an e-mail confirming that I had been accepted for this elective among only 50 other students. I then set to work immediately organising my departure. After overcoming several logistical challenges, I was able to travel to my destination in the United Kingdom in what was my first trip abroad. I arrived at Oxford University and lodged at the John Radcliffe Hospital for 10 weeks, where I joined local medical students in their cardiovascular and plastic and reconstructive surgery rotations.

Top tips

1. Try to choose a country where you would like to specialise in; an elective could be a step on the road of your future specialty.
2. Try to make contact with as many people as possible; they will help you acclimatise to the environment rapidly and effectively.
3. Ask your mentor politely to be involved in his/her research work; the elective is a very good opportunity to participate in a research project – aim for an output of some sort; a published case report is a very good achievement.
4. Do not push yourself to attend all day in the hospital. Elective is also a time for sightseeing and having fun!
5. Document everything, by either taking photos or recording videos or writing down your daily diary, and present it to your colleagues – it is essential to share knowledge when you return.

During the first days of my elective, I experienced the so-called cultural shock. Everything in the city and its hospitals seemed close to perfection – a far cry from what I was familiar with in my home city. The quality of health service was extraordinary, and I initially felt a little out of my depth. This was not because I was unfamiliar with the knowledge, but rather due to the highly organised and systematic way in which it was applied and the structured division of labour which characterised the hospital environment. Fortunately, my training was free, and I was able to access a range of facilities including wards, clinics, operation theatres, libraries and lecture theatres. I saw for the first time a state-of-the-art robotic surgical system and participated in daily ward rounds and bedside teaching with prominent clinicians.

My experience at Oxford was incredibly enriching, I hope to return in the future and participate in clinical research. I still maintain contact with former students and doctors at Oxford to this day.

Obstetrics and gynaecology, Dakar, Senegal

Ira Kleine

My elective planning started with a simple wish list: (1) exposure to obstetrics and gynaecology in a low-resource setting and (2) improve my fluency in conversational and medical French. *Le résultat*: Dakar, Senegal, with specialisation in obstetric fistulas.

No amount of reading on health systems or epidemiology compares to seeing first-hand the difficulties that arise from sparse resources and out-of-pocket health expenditure, as well as the cultural attitudes to health that ensue. The stories of women and girls being treated for obstetric fistulas epitomised this struggle: lack of antenatal care, midwife-less homebirths and prolonged obstructed labour (up to 9 days!), followed by emergency caesarean section, stillbirth, fistula, urinary incontinence, social exclusion and even divorce. The experience was incredibly eye opening, giving me unique insight into the country's healthcare challenges, huge respect for the local doctors and an even greater appreciation for the NHS. Moreover, travelling alone in a country where English is not widely spoken was a sink-or-swim linguistic experience – the perfect (albeit exhausting) environment for fast improvement.

Eight months before lift-off, having already spent months planning my dream elective and securing funding, the first hurdle hit: Ebola. I stubbornly decided to gamble my chances and breathed a huge sigh of relief, alongside all Senegalese, when the country was declared Ebola-free. While on placement, the fatal consequences of out-of-pocket health expenditure and waste of precious resources due to lack of clinical protocols (e.g. lack of blood transfusion monitoring) were frustrating and emotionally draining, magnified by not having a companion of similar background to debrief with. However, the latter – loneliness – was perhaps my greatest challenge. I got to know many amazing people, but yearned for the familiarity of being able to chat freely, without a language barrier, to a close friend. It also made me feel very vulnerable. I was highly aware of the daily dangers (e.g. non-roadworthy, seatbelt-less cars) and the fragility of my own existence, exacerbated by the fatalistic attitude to life and death held by those around me – understandable when resources are not available to treat; my own prolonged diarrhoeal illness while on elective did not help either.

My experience resulted in a change of career goals, as I realised that living and working in a low-resource environment is not for me. It really is impossible to know how you will react to the challenging situations that arise. So, my greatest advice to you is go try it for yourself! (But take a friend.)

Perspective of an elective host

William Tamale

As an HIV/AIDS specialist in Uganda, I see on average 20–25 HIV patients on anti-retroviral therapy per day. Alongside my clinical work, I manage the clinic and run clinical trials – roughly one every 2 years. Accordingly, I receive great interest from overseas elective students who want to learn more about the clinical situation faced by doctors and patients in a lower-resource setting like Uganda. To date, I have supervised over 30 elective medical students from the United States, the United Kingdom, Netherlands, Kenya and Nigeria.

As a host doctor, I am intrigued and excited about our elective students. Particularly, given that you are soon to become doctors faced with patients who depend on your clinical skills and judgement to solve medical and social problems. An elective serves as an ideal opportunity to begin that transition – from student to practitioner. While many of my elective students have been enthusiastic and engaging, I have witnessed some who do not pay sufficient attention. This is a great pity. The skills you acquire through medical training and your elective will define you as a doctor – from your medical competency to the impression you leave with clients and patients.

Reflecting on your quality as a doctor and insisting on its improvement is key. I regularly seek feedback from my patients, who have expectations too. Bear this in mind when you arrive on elective: medicine is a two-way process. Do not be afraid to examine and communicate – eyeballing a patient is not adequate; use the full clinical skills you have been equipped with, be they percussion or auscultation. Wherever you are coming from, in this part of the world, clinical acumen remains central to decision-making. Your generation of doctors can play a role in respecting and nurturing these clinical skills and competencies – which I believe are central to the doctor–patient relationship.

Research requires doctors who are trustworthy, patient and knowledgeable. If you have these attributes as a medical student – hold on to them. In doing research, always look to contribute meaningfully to the body of information out there. Clinical trials are slow and take years to run. Further, they depend on your relationship with the patient and this is what is so important about the elective: you will see people not numbers.

Finally, I encourage you to develop and maintain empathy for your future patients. Best of luck for your electives.

Weebale Nyo!

CHAPTER 6

Further degrees

CONTENTS

DIPLOMA

Daniel Di Francesco

What is a diploma?

Depending on where and who you are, a diploma can mean many things – you might earn the qualification at a school, college or university. For medical students (and qualified doctors) in the United Kingdom, the postgraduate diploma or PGDip will be your focus. These courses are typically less intensive than a full master's degree, but although they contain fewer topics, those covered are often at comparable depth. As the UK PGDip does not translate well to other countries – this chapter will offer an overview and guidance on diplomas for medical students based in the United Kingdom.

Diploma: Deciding
Why?

While you may already have quite a lot on your academic plate, a diploma offers medical students the chance to study more niche subjects in greater detail, without necessarily requiring an interruption or intercalation in their medical studies. You might want to gain specific practical skills or improve your career prospects by demonstrating above and beyond commitment to a specific area.

What?

There are myriad opportunities to undertake a diploma; however, note that some of these are not available to medical students. Diplomas usually come as two components: the course and the exam. To be eligible for the exam, candidates must complete the course. Course completion will require a high level of attendance and the timely submission of any coursework. The content of courses will vary considerably depending on the type of diploma you take. Some may include practical elements and field trips; others will be solely lecture based. Table 6.1 summarises some of the most popular courses available. Even if you cannot undertake a course during your medical degree, it is never too early to start thinking about your career ambitions and what qualifications will support them.

When?

If you are keen on studying one of the diplomas open to medical students, it is important to get the timing right. Consider your other commitments: In your first year, you will most likely need time to find your feet studying medicine; while in your final year, you may be stressed and time pressed revising for final exams. Many medical students wait until graduation before pursuing a diploma. This increases not only the number of courses available to you, but also the likelihood your diploma will be compatible with your future career aims. That said, unlike higher degrees discussed elsewhere in this chapter – the diploma is a chance to build a wider knowledge base and is only rarely viewed as a requirement for a given career route.

Diploma: Doing

Selecting a course

The first step will be to research your chosen diploma in detail. Broadly, your options are medical, medically related or non-medical courses. Because these courses are so specialised, it is important to find one that offers modules compatible with your interests. Nearly all courses nowadays offer a good level of detail on their website, but you can also request a prospectus or contact the university or college directly for specific questions. Pay particular attention to the contact hours, some may require on-site attendance while others may offer distance learning and online modules. Finally, consider the location and cost of the course itself and whether this will be sustainable alongside travel, textbooks and other course expenses. You should remember that bursaries and extra funding are the exception rather than the rule, as most of those undertaking a diploma will already be in employment.

Forward strategy

A diploma is particularly helpful at enabling you to gain experience in areas you have no previous academic grounding in. For example, you may wish to do a diploma in a field unrelated to medicine – such as economics or politics. A 1-year PGDip would be an ideal way to build knowledge in this area – similar to an intercalated bachelor degree. However, applying for these courses would require you to have an honours degree and so could only be done after an intercalated degree, necessitating another interruption of your medical studies. However, if you are set on becoming a leader in health economics – this approach could set you apart from the crowd. Develop a strategy and test out your options and their feasibility with a mentor or your medical programme director. It is worth considering the type of institution offering the diploma and what kind of accreditation it has received. Reputable institutions will offer diplomas which are nationally or internationally recognised.

Completing a course

How the course is taught will vary greatly so it is worth researching this in detail, either by visiting the course directors or speaking to previous students. Some will be based around online learning modules and an Multiple Choice Question (MCQ) exam paper, while the more intensive courses will require clinical tasks and essays or OSCE-style examinations. While diplomas are much less likely to involve research and potential publications than master's degrees, there will still be plenty of opportunities to take advantage of. Build a relationship with the course lecturers or conveners who are likely to be experts in their field; network with your colleagues including those more senior or at advanced stages of their training – you may be one of only a few medical students; and finally, maintain contact with your colleagues once the diploma is finished should further opportunities for collaboration arise. At the very least, you could consider writing a reflective report of your experience on the course to publish online or in print.

Conclusion

A diploma can serve as a great opportunity for medical students and doctors to broaden their professional knowledge, experience and networks without the cost and time requirements of undertaking a full degree. However, deciding which course to take should be informed by a clear set of objectives – whether this is developing a clinical skill, gaining new knowledge or building connections with others in a given field. If you are confident the course can deliver – then it will be worth the investment.

Pros

- Learn from specialists about an area of particular interest to you
- Acquire practical skills
- Meet other clinicians interested in your field
- Strengthen your job application

Cons

- Financial cost
- Time commitment

Common pitfalls

1. *Time management.*

   It is easy to underestimate the time commitment and stress of taking up additional courses – you have to remember that your medical degree should be your main priority. Bear in mind that you may sign up to something at the start of the year when the workload is light, but you are committing to working right up until exam season.

2. *Right reasons.*

   A diploma does not offer any points on the UK foundation programme application like an intercalated degree does, and it is by no means an instant pass to a job in your chosen field. It is important to take an extra qualification for the right reasons; if it is an area that truly interests you, it will be much easier to motivate yourself and put in the necessary hours.

3. *Right time.*

   If you are making a year-long commitment, you should think carefully about what the demands on your time will be from start to finish. For most, the best years will be the second to fourth of the standard medical degree, since you will be settled and will not have finals bearing down on you.

Further reading

Burrard-Lucas, N. Clinical diplomas. *GP Online.* 2014. http://www.gponline.com/clinical-diplomas/article/1287148. Accessed on June 14, 2017.

Davies, C. Diploma in tropical medicine and hygiene. *BMJ Careers.* 2009. http://careers.bmj.com/careers/advice/Diploma_in_Tropical_Medicine_and_Hygiene. Accessed on June 14, 2017.

Patel, S. Postgraduate qualifications. *BMJ Careers.* 2009. http://careers.bmj.com/careers/advice/view-article.html?id=20000042. Accessed on June 14, 2017.

Table 6.1 Popular diploma courses in the United Kingdom

Diploma	Awarded by	Course content	Cost	Medical student friendly?	Notes	More info
Diploma in philosophy of medicine/diploma in history of medicine/diploma in medical care of conflict and catastrophes	The Worshipful Society of Apothecaries of London	One year – Saturday lectures; two exam papers and dissertation	£800 (£562.50 for medical students)	Yes – weekend study and student discount. King's College funds two places per year	Popular with students and doctors. Less career-focussed	Society of Apothecaries (http://www.apothecaries.org/)
Diploma in tropical medicine and hygiene	London School of Hygiene and Tropical Medicine	Three months full time – lectures, seminars, lab work	£6350	No – requires a medical qualification and preferably 3 years of clinical experience	Highly regarded. Necessary requirement to work with Médecins Sans Frontières (MSF)	London School of Hygiene and Tropical Medicine (http://www.lshtm.ac.uk/study/cpd/stmh.html#second)
Diploma in tropical medicine and hygiene	Liverpool School of Tropical Medicine	Thirteen weeks full time – lectures, tutorials, seminars, practicals	£6000	No – requires a medical qualification and preferably 2 years of clinical experience	Highly regarded. Necessary requirement to work with MSF	Liverpool School of Tropical Medicine (http://www.lstmed.ac.uk/study/courses/diploma-in-tropical-medicine-hygiene)

(Continued)

Table 6.1 (Continued) Popular diploma courses in the United Kingdom

Diploma	Awarded by	Course content	Cost	Medical student friendly?	Notes	More info
Training/general practitioner-focused diplomas						
Diploma of the Royal College of Obstetricians and Gynaecologists (DRCOG)	Royal College of Obstetricians and Gynaecologists	Two exam papers	£408	No – requires General Medical Council (GMC) registration		Obstetrics and Gynaecology (http://www.rcog.org.uk /education-and-exams /examinations/diploma)
Diploma in Geriatric Medicine (DGM)	Royal College of Physicians	Written and clinical examination	£570	No – requires medical degree and 2 years' experience		Geriatric Medicine (http:// www.rcplondon.ac.uk /medical-careers-training /postgraduate-exams /diploma-geriatric -medicine)
Diploma in Occupational Medicine (DOccMed)	Faculty of Occupational Medicine	Written and oral examination and portfolio assessment	£1128	No – requires medical degree		Faculty of Occupational Medicine (http://www .fom.ac.uk/education /examinations/diplomas /doccmed)

(Continued)

Table 6.1 (Continued)   Popular diploma courses in the United Kingdom

Diploma	Awarded by	Course content	Cost	Medical student friendly?	Notes	More info
Diploma of the Faculty of Sexual and Reproductive Healthcare (DFSRH)	Royal College of Obstetricians and Gynaecologists	Online assessment, assessed workshops and clinical experience	£125 plus local training costs	No – requires medical degree		Faculty of Sexual and Reproductive Healthcare (http://www.fsrh.org /pages/Diploma_of_the _FSRH.asp)
Diploma in Otolaryngology – Head and Neck Surgery (DO-HNS)	Royal College of Surgeons	Written paper and Objective Structured Clinical Examination (OSCE)	£1540	No – requires medical degree		Otolaryngology (http:// www.rcseng.ac.uk /exams/surgical/dohns)

Note: Accurate as of 2016.

INTERCALATED BACHELOR'S AND MASTER'S DEGREES

Jonathan C. H. Lau

Introduction

One way to enhance your time at medical school is to undertake an additional year of study that culminates in the award of a bachelor's degree or in some cases a master's degree. These so-called intercalated degrees provide a unique opportunity for students to learn more about a subject of their choice in far greater depth than would otherwise be possible as part of their standard medical course. The aim of this section is to describe what intercalated degrees involve and how they may be used to benefit you as much as possible.

Basics

Studying for an intercalated degree involves an additional year of full-time study on top of your core medical programme. In some institutions, such as Nottingham, University College London (UCL), Oxford and Cambridge, which offer a compulsory six-year course, this comes as no choice. However, in others which offer the ordinary 5-year programme, the option to pursue an intercalated degree may be taken after the second, third or fourth year of study.

The choices of subjects on offer are broad and can vary further from institution to institution. However, while most options enable you to focus on one specific area of medicine such as immunology, neuroscience or physiology, it is also possible for you to stray further from the basic sciences and pursue subjects such as philosophy, history or even management studies. Most choices culminate in the award of a so-called intercalated bachelor's degree; while less commonly, some lead to an intercalated master's degree, but these tend to be clinically orientated and, hence, may only be taken by students who have spent at least one year of study in clinics (i.e. years 3, 4 or higher). Nevertheless, irrespective of their final award title, as intercalated degrees, both bachelor's and master's courses have the same format and structure of learning.

Details

The intercalated year differs from the standard medical course in a few key areas. First, the teaching tends to be less structured and more flexible. A number of optional modules may be taken to suit particular interests within your chosen subject, and as a result, not all given lectures and seminars have to be attended, but that does not stop you from going to them if you wish! Second, assessment takes the form of essay writing, as you will be asked questions that make you think critically about your subject and encourage you to have a dialogue. This is likely to come as a surprise to those who may not have written an essay since leaving school and/or sitting medical entrance exams such as the Biomedical Admissions Test (BMAT). Finally, you will have to participate in a research or library project and put your findings into a lengthy dissertation (~5000–10,000 words), which is usually submitted towards the end of the year. The research component is valuable for a number of reasons, not least because it encourages you to become your own 'expert' in a particular field. It also allows you, at a very early stage, to engage in research activities, which can help inform your interests for the future (e.g. whether you wish to go into academia or conduct research in a lab or another setting), not to mention having a chance to get a paper published.

Why do one?

It is important to take some time to decide whether you want to undertake an intercalated BSc in the first place, before you make any decision about the subject and where you wish to study. While it is becoming increasingly commonplace for medical students who want to go into research and academia to intercalate, this is not absolutely necessary, and indeed, many may simply wish to take an extra year for the sake of learning more about a topic or provide themselves with a backup option in case they fail to qualify or choose to leave medicine at the end of their course; all of which are acceptable reasons to take a year out. Nonetheless, research conducted on behalf of graduating medical students have found that those who finished medical school with an intercalated degree possessed deeper analytical skills and strategic styles of learning than those who did not. Moreover, people who intercalate have an opportunity to get their research published, which can help strengthen their applications for future jobs, irrespective of wanting to spend time in academia. In addition, having an intercalated degree is prerequisite for those wishing to join combined MB–PhD programmes.

Where to go

The choice of where to spend your intercalated year is interesting as few medical schools allow for such 'branching' decisions to be made. Schools that offer 6-year programmes with compulsory intercalated degrees tend to have very strict policies preventing its students from leaving their own institutions to intercalate. However, if the opportunity is available to you, it may be useful to think about going to a different university. While some institutions may exclusively offer certain subjects, others may offer the same or similar courses but with additional opportunities. It goes without saying that increased levels of competition are to be expected, but this should not be an issue if you are convinced that a change of scenery, in line with your academic pursuits, are worth the decision to study elsewhere.

Succeeding

Once you have embarked on your programme of choice at your chosen institution, you should feel like every other undergraduate student on campus, the stress of trying to achieve a good result at the end of the year, namely, a 2:1 condition or higher, pressing on your mind! As alluded to earlier, one of the biggest difficulties will be adjusting to the change in teaching style, notably, the requirement to write essays for the majority, if not all, of your exams. From the very beginning, it is important to understand the broader implications of what you are being taught rather than simply absorb the knowledge as facts, which is what many medical students become very used to, particularly during the first two years of study. Remember that your chosen subject will be taught up to the limits of what is currently known so it should become clear that for every question set, there is likely to be no right or wrong answer, instead, only ample room for discussion (as opposed to regurgitation). It is important to be proactive with your learning during your intercalated year and encourage yourself to read widely around your lectures, avoid relying on textbooks and instead start reading journal papers and reviews or ask lecturers for their opinions on matters that you find interesting.

Another useful tip for success is to ensure that you pick a good research project for your dissertation or laboratory-based research. A common mistake is for students to pick projects that sound interesting without necessarily going into the details of what is involved. Here, it is important to speak to the supervisor in charge face to face, before making a final decision. This will help you to avoid easy but risky traps such as poor projects. During your intercalated year, you will be exposed to research and may start to feel drawn to it, particularly if you are working on the side of a laboratory. This comes naturally and may prompt some to consider applying for an MB-PhD or some other form of postgraduate degree (e.g. a research master's), as covered in the next chapter.

Conclusion

It goes without saying that studying for an extra year means incurring additional financial costs while also prolonging the time it takes to qualify. Consequently, such drawbacks to pursuing an intercalated degree need to be carefully considered as well. Some take the view that intercalated degrees prevent them from seeing patients as soon or as much as possible while at medical school. Meanwhile, others feel that these disadvantages are overwhelmingly offset by the diverse potential opportunities of an intercalated degree. Getting used to a different style of learning may also be seen as off-putting, particularly if the intercalated degree only lasts for a year relative to the entire length of the standard course. I would argue that while the intercalated degree undoubtedly demands and expects a fair amount of your time and investment, the benefits tangibly outweigh the disadvantages in that it offers a change of perspective which is especially valuable. This comes at a time when a greater appreciation and awareness of scientific research, evidence-based techniques and the limits of our knowledge in various fields is becoming more important.

Further reading

Barnett-Vanes, A., and Shalhoub, J. Studying for an intercalated BSc externally. *Student BMJ* 2014;22:g2194.

Gardner, K., and Olojugba, C. Should I do an intercalated BSc? *Student BMJ* 2008;16:238–9.

Intercalate.co.uk. http://intercalate.co.uk/.

Leung, W. Is studying for an intercalated degree a wise career move? *Student BMJ* 2001;9:418–9.

McManus, C. To BSc or not to BSc. . . . *Student BMJ* 2011;19:d7559. doi:10.1136/sbmj.d7559.

PhD

Ada E. D. Teo

Background

A PhD, or doctor of philosophy, is an advanced postgraduate degree that usually involves at least 3 years of independent research on an original topic, culminating in the conferment of the title 'doctor' in academia.

Coupling a PhD with your medical degree allows both immediate gratification from patient interaction and long-term benefits of medical innovation. A PhD in medicine will be able to quench your thirst for knowledge underlying the whys and hows of disease pathophysiology, with the potential for translation into novel therapies. In addition, the scientific rigour of a PhD will train you to think more critically about new treatments, analyse evidence and evaluate clinical trials as a clinician-scientist.

As the journey to becoming a consultant requires at least a decade, it is understandable that most medical students are eager to start their practice and climb the ladder as quickly as possible. As such, the thought of taking at least another 3 years away from medicine to do a PhD may seem unappealing. But being trained in both science and medicine, clinician-scientists can pursue a wider variety of opportunities including – but definitely not limited to – clinical practice, teaching, pharmaceutical industries, university or departmental administration. The opportunities are endless. The power of clinical insight allows the fluid movement of clinician-scientists across the research and clinical arenas. Being adept at more than one language also makes you uniquely qualified to lead large, collaborative teams. Alternatively, clinician-scientists may choose more non-traditional career options such as consulting, global health or policy-making. Whatever route you desire, this synergy will give you a unique advantage in shaping a career that matches all your interests.

Timing

As with many other aspects of a medical career, there is no ideal time for a PhD. Many universities in the United States and several in the United Kingdom and across Europe offer a formal intercalated MD–PhD or MB–PhD programme where the 3–4 research years are intertwined with the normal clinical curriculum to ensure the continuation of clinical work during the research period. Alternative options are to either intercalate a self-organised PhD or defer your PhD until post-graduation.

Undertaking a PhD early (before completion of your medical degree) will be less of a burden financially as you are unlikely to be paying off housing debts or be in the midst of setting up your own family. Starting early will also give you more time to build your portfolio in research, and attaining the PhD will certainly give you an edge in getting your first-choice specialty. On the other hand, embarking on a PhD at a later stage (after specialisation) means that you can tailor your PhD topic according to your clinical specialty as you may have a better idea of what your long-term medical career may look like.

However, it would be immensely more difficult to secure time out from specialty training and put your medical job and steady income on hold to pursue a higher degree. In these cases, retaining some clinical work is up to you; covering a hospital shift from time to time can help to keep your skills updated and, in some cases, be of significant financial help. Furthermore, maintaining some clinical work can also help you keep a focus on the importance of research in the path to becoming a consultant. That being said, it is important to note that many funding bodies may limit the amount of time allowed in the clinical setting.

Your PhD subject

In a nutshell, you can do your PhD in any area, be it a natural or social science. Most clinician-scientists earn their PhDs in biomedical disciplines such as biochemistry, genetics, immunology, neuroscience or pharmacology, just to name a few. Others choose to explore areas beyond laboratory disciplines, including anthropology, computational biology, epidemiology, health economics and policy, history of medicine or even sociology.

Unless your institution or funding body stipulates certain requirements on the field of study, there is no rule as to what subject you should pursue. Through a PhD, you are seeking to master the scientific method and experience the rigour of critical thinking. Many who already have an area of specialty in mind opt to do their PhDs in the same area, or think that it is a must. This is not necessary, especially if you are considering an intercalated MB–PhD programme where the research is midway in your medical degree. Upon attaining your medical qualifications, the field of research would have already moved on. You should view the PhD as a lesson in persistence, creative original thought and, last but not least, time management. Skills acquired from the experience, be it interpersonal, statistical, writing, or presenting skills, are all invaluable and transferable.

Organising a PhD

You could arrange your PhD within the university where you are studying for your medical degree or independently with organisations or research charities. Committing yourself to a higher degree and the further years it may take, choosing a topic of research and obtaining funding may seem overwhelming initially. Application to the degree programme and grant writing should begin at least one year in advance, but your PhD supervisor will have some experience in seeking funding. Established supervisors may already have some ongoing funding, either from the university, local research bursaries or charitable organisations and may not require your input into the grant application process. Make sure you check with your supervisor prior to PhD commencement what arrangements are in place and if any action needs to be taken on your part.

Your supervisor will be the person you interact with regularly for at least three straight years and not only will they have a pivotal role in your project, but also their influence on the rest of your career may be considerable. Key questions to ask are as follows: Do you like their supervisory/advising style and personality? Do they manage the lab well? Do they encourage more junior PhD students to present their work at meetings? And most importantly, can you see yourselves getting along and having meaningful discussions for 3+ years? Often, in the search for a suitable PhD supervisor, one tends to focus too much on publication track record and impact factor; of course, the quality of research your

Five top tips

1. *Decide on a reference manager early on (EndNote, Mendeley etc.) and organise your readings.*
   Research the different features that each reference manager software offers and more importantly, find out what the rest of your lab uses. This will make it much easier to highlight articles and share citations within your group.
2. *Set up regular notifications on PubMed based on keywords.*
   In order to keep updated on the latest articles published in your area, it is crucial to sign up to daily or weekly notifications on PubMed based on keywords or phrases in your field.
3. *Keep an open mind – be flexible about your research topic.*
   The importance of keeping an open mind about the area of research and labs to join for your PhD cannot be overemphasised. Many students come in thinking they know exactly what they want to do for their PhD and consequently restrict themselves and their scope of work. By casting a wide net and considering a variety of opportunities, you may just surprise yourself by embarking on a different research direction than you had originally envisioned.
4. *Present at as many conferences as possible.*
   Although most PhD projects last at least 3 years, and you may not obtain final results or make any conclusions until the end of this time, interim findings can be submitted to national or international meetings, and your supervisor should encourage you to do so.

5. *Understand that embarking on a PhD extends an already-long medical degree, so make sure you are committed to this journey and its time frame.*

Remaining patient, persistent and tenacious is key to succeeding in your PhD and at the same time, enjoying the process. Of these, patience might be the most rewarding, as procedures and setup may be much slower than in the clinical arena, especially if you are embarking on a new project with no research infrastructure already in place.

supervisor works on is crucial, but more importantly, will you integrate well into the lab and use the resources available to set yourself up for a successful PhD?

Conclusion

Choose to do a PhD for the right reasons. Ultimately, an MB–PhD would not be a good fit if you saw it merely as a means to an end (e.g. just for a better chance of getting into the specialty you desire), so commit to it only if you harbour a genuine thirst for knowledge and passion for research. A PhD can open many doors for your medical career, but what you do post-PhD is equally important – only by keeping abreast of updates in your field of research and by maintaining relationships formed during your PhD will you benefit from all the doors it opens.

Further reading

Barnett-Vanes, A. and Allen, R. *How to Complete a PhD in the Medical and Clinical Sciences.* Wiley–Blackwell, Hoboken, NJ, 2017.

Barnett-Vanes, A., Ho, G. and Cox, T. M. Clinician-scientist MB/PhD training in the UK: A nationwide survey of medical school policy. *BMJ Open.* 2015;5(12):e009852. doi:10.1136/bmjopen-2015-009852.

Schwartz, M. A. The importance of stupidity in scientific research. *J. Cell Sci.* 2008;121:1771.

Schwartz, M. A. The importance of indifference in scientific research. *J. Cell Sci.* 2015;128(15):2745–6.

MPH

Jason Sarfo-Annin

Background

A Master of Public Health (MPH) is a specialist multidisciplinary programme aimed at postgraduates, focussed on improving the health of communities and populations. It is designed to develop individuals in the practice of public health as opposed to public health master of philosophy degree programmes that train in research methods.

Typical programme content

The content of a MPH programme can vary considerably depending on where you study. In the United Kingdom, public health registrars are usually expected to obtain an MPH during training. Consequently, many UK courses are aligned to the content of the Faculty of Public Health curriculum [1] and designed to help prepare candidates to pass the Part A examination of the Membership of the Faculty of Public Health. In the United States, courses are designed to meet the accreditation requirements of the Council on Education for Public Health [2]. Broadly speaking, most programmes are typically 1 year in length and have both mandatory and optional courses – see Table 6.2 for the five core public health disciplines and example course titles. There are MPH programmes that are built with a dedicated focus or concentration, e.g. nutrition public health. Furthermore, there are master's programmes labelled as an MSc or MA that have similar content to a MPH and have equivalence.

Deciding where to do it

After eligibility, the two most important factors should be the programme content and the cost. If you have an interest in an area such as environmental health MPH programmes that focus on the field, or provide the option to take modules on the field, should be ranking high in your shortlist. Some programmes provide more course choice than others, and if your interests lie in multiple areas, this may be beneficial.

Table 6.2 Core public health disciplines

Discipline	Explanation	Example course titles
Biostatistics	Concepts and practice of statistical analysis to investigate problems related to health	• Applied Regression Analysis • Fundamentals of Clinical Trials • Analysis of Categorical Data • Probability and Statistical Inference
Epidemiology	Study of the distribution and determinants of disability or disease in population groups	• Public Health Surveillance Design • Analysis of Longitudinal Data • Epidemiology of Malaria • Measurement Issues in Chronic Disease Epidemiology
Health services administration (policy and management)	Multidisciplinary field concerned with the delivery, quality and costs of healthcare for individuals and populations	• Organisational Management • Public Financing of Healthcare • Economic Evaluation of Healthcare Programmes • Public Health Law
Social and behavioural sciences	Behavioural, social and cultural factors related to individual and population health and health disparities	• Social Determinants of Health Inequalities • Race and Health • Substance Abuse and Addiction • Qualitative Research Methods
Environmental health sciences	Identification and control of biological, physical and chemical factors in the natural environment which affect health	• Public Health Toxicology • Climate Change and Health • Injury Prevention and Control • Public Health Emergency Preparedness and Response

Table 6.3 provides a non-exhaustive list of 1-year general MPH courses in the United Kingdom. There are many more that have a dedicated focus. A non-exhaustive list of European public health departments can be found via the Association of Schools of Public Health in the European Region (see the 'Further reading' section). Highly regarded European public health programmes outside the United Kingdom include Erasmus University in Rotterdam, the University of Copenhagen and the Karolinska Institutet in Sweden.

Many highly regarded schools of public health are based in the United States. Along with well-known names such as Harvard and Johns Hopkins, institutions such as the University of North Carolina at Chapel Hill and Emory University in Atlanta have alumni in many national departments of health and international bodies such as the WHO. Information on US courses can be found via the Schools and Programs of Public Health Program Finder (see the 'Further reading' section).

Course structure and funding

The benefit of studying in the United States is that the academic credit system enables students to take courses from other university departments such as law, business or government. Most courses in the United States have a mandatory practical component that entails working for an organisation which may be in the private or public sector. Most courses in the United Kingdom require a dissertation. In the United Kingdom, the benchmark for tuition fees, as of 2016/2017 is around £9000 for UK students. There are courses which charge less, and some institutions provide the option of distance learning which can lower the financial burden. The tuition fees for a MPH in the United States are usually in excess of $30,000 and roughly double this amount at universities such as Johns Hopkins and Harvard. However, not all courses have such eye-watering figures. A degree in Sweden or Denmark is currently tuition fee free to all European Union (EU) nationals; see the 'Further reading' section for funding options.

How to organise it

Few courses explicitly allow intercalating students, as an MPH is aimed at postgraduates or those with years of practical experience. Although most programmes allow entry if you have already intercalated, some may accept students without a bachelor's degree if they have enough related experience that can be evidenced (if in doubt, contact the course administrator). As most programmes are pre-built courses, you will need to go through an application procedure external to your medical school. Note also that postgraduate programme term dates vary between institutions and may not coincide with your medical school programme; therefore, you may need to apply for academic leave of absence. If the course fits your interests well but does not allow intercalation, it may be worth considering enrolling after medical school graduation, either immediately before, during or after postgraduate training.

Pros/cons

Advantages

- *Diversity of students:* Many students travel from around the world to study an MPH in Europe or North America. You learn just as much from your peers as you do from professors.
- *Multidisciplinary learning:* The ability to cover disciplines such as economics, law, business, management and politics provides a view of the role of health and healthcare in society that is not taught at medical school.
- *Enhancing basic research competencies:* The biostatistics and epidemiology covered in the course is in much more depth than those covered at medical school and provides good grounding for a career in academic medicine.
- *Time away from medical school:* Looking at health as a concept for populations rather than individuals may give you a better sense of what your career goals are and how to plan for them.

Disadvantages

- *Experience:* Many courses assume prior practical experience and use this to drive discussion and learning. Medical students can find aspects of an MPH programme challenging.
- *Knowledge transferability:* Depending on where you study and the focus of the programme, some courses may be centred on navigating health systems that work very differently to your own.
- *Breadth as opposed to depth:* Given the short time frame and numerous disciplines covered, many MPH students leave with a sense of unfinished business.
- *Language:* Although many European universities offer courses in English, integrating into the local community can be difficult without basic fluency in the native language.

Future career impact

An MPH programme provides some grounding for a career in academic medicine, whether that be in clinical research or specifically in public health. Master level degrees usually provide more short-listing points at foundation and speciality training applications than an intercalated bachelor's degree. Additionally, should you wish to become a public health trainee, having an MPH can give you the option to shorten your training time. A relatively new and popular doctoral-level qualification, the Doctor of Public Health (DrPH) is aimed at training for leadership roles in public health. It usually requires an MPH prior to entry. With the appropriate experience, an MPH can provide a route to a wide variety of employment opportunities in roles aligned to healthcare. Ranging from non-profit charity and advocacy groups to private organisations such as consultancy firms, local government or public health departments to large international organisations such as the World Bank.

Conclusion

The MPH programme provides the tools for individuals to improve the health of populations, as opposed to medical school which focusses primarily on the health of individuals. Opportunities to develop knowledge and skills in areas such as quantitative methods and healthcare management can provide significant added value to a medical degree and career within or outside clinical medicine.

Top tips and common pitfalls

1. *Plan very early – at least 18 months before the start of the course.*

    a. Scholarship applications are often labour intensive and tend to have application deadlines 9–12 months before the academic year in question.

    b. Some universities have entrance exams, e.g. the Graduate Record Examination in the United States.

2. *Is this course right for you?*

    a. A Master of Business Administration (MBA) or a Master of Public Policy (MPP) degree may be better suited to your interests if management or policy disciplines interest you most. You will usually need to wait until you have graduated from medical school to apply for these programmes. Take the time to research the programmes available and speak to people who have completed them.

3. *Funding*

    a. The most common barrier to studying an MPH is financial viability, particularly in US or European cities with a high cost of living. Many universities have dedicated scholarships with a wide range of eligibility criteria. There are also many external awards available.

    b. Remember that every little bit helps; multiple scholarships or awards providing smaller financial grants may be a more practical and fruitful route of funding than a highly competitive award that covers all or the majority of the financial cost.

References

1. Faculty of Public Health. *Specialty Training.* http://www.fph.org.uk /specialty_training. Accessed on June 26, 2017.

2. Council on Education for Public Health. http://ceph.org/. Accessed on June 26, 2017.

Further reading

MPH programme finder resources:

Association of Schools of Public Health in the European Region. http://www .aspher.org/.

Royal Medical Benevolent Fund. *Intercalated degrees.* http://rmbf.org/medical -students/intercalated-degrees/.

Schools and Programs of Public Health. http://sophas.org/program-finder/.

Student Doctor Network. http://forums.studentdoctor.net/forums/public-health -degrees-masters-and-doctoral.94/.

Financial resources:

For international students applying to courses in the United States: Fulbright Foreign Student Program: https://exchanges.state.gov/non-us/program/fulbright -foreign-student-program.

For information on funding an intercalated degree or master's as a UK medical student: http://www.money4medstudents.org/intercalated-degrees.

Scholarships for international students applying to courses in the United Kingdom: Chevening Scholarship: http://www.chevening.org/.

Table 6.3 General UK MPH programmes

Institution	Degree awarded	Optional modules	Dissertation	Explicitly allow intercalating students?	Website
University of Aberdeen	MPH	Yes	Standard or extended project		https://www.abdn.ac.uk/study/postgraduate-taught/degree-programmes/909/master-of-public-health/
Anglia Ruskin University	MSc in public health	No	Yes		http://www.anglia.ac.uk/study/postgraduate/public-health
Barts and the London School of Medicine and Dentistry	MSc in public health	Yes	Yes		http://www.icms.qmul.ac.uk/chs/education/postgrad/msc_pgdip_public_health/
University of Bedfordshire	MSc in public health	No	Yes		https://www.beds.ac.uk/howtoapply/courses/postgraduate/next-year/public-health2
University of Birmingham	MPH	Yes	Yes		http://www.birmingham.ac.uk/postgraduate/courses/taught/med/public-health.aspx
Birmingham City University	MSc in public health	No	Yes		http://www.bcu.ac.uk/courses/public-health
Bournemouth University	MSc in public health	No	Yes		https://www1.bournemouth.ac.uk/study/courses/msc-public-health

(*Continued*)

Table 6.3 (Continued)   General UK MPH programmes

Institution	Degree awarded	Optional modules	Dissertation	Explicitly allow intercalating students?	Website
University of Bradford	MPH	Yes	Yes		http://www.bradford.ac.uk/study/courses/info/public-health-mph
Brighton and Sussex Medical School	MSc in public health	Yes	Yes	Yes	https://www.bsms.ac.uk/postgraduate/taught-degrees/public-health.aspx
University of Cardiff	MPH	Yes	Yes		http://www.cardiff.ac.uk/study/postgraduate/taught/courses/course/public-health-mph
University of Chester	MPH	Yes	Yes		https://www1.chester.ac.uk/postgraduate/master-public-health?mode=2095
City University	MPH	No	Yes		http://www.city.ac.uk/courses/postgraduate/masters-in-public-health-mph
University of Derby	MPH	Yes	No		http://www.derby.ac.uk/courses/postgraduate/public-health-masters/
University of Dundee	MPH	Yes	Yes		http://www.dundee.ac.uk/study/pg/public-health/
University of Edinburgh	MPH	Yes	Yes		http://www.ed.ac.uk/molecular-genetic-population/mph

(Continued)

Table 6.3 (Continued) General UK MPH programmes

Institution	Degree awarded	Optional modules	Dissertation	Explicitly allow intercalating students?	Website
University of Glasgow	MPH	Yes	Yes		http://www.gla.ac.uk/postgraduate/taught /publichealth/
Glasgow Caledonian University	MSc in Public Health	Yes	Yes		http://www.gcu.ac.uk/study/postgraduate /courses/
Imperial College London	MPH	Yes	Yes		https://www.imperial.ac.uk/medicine /study/postgraduate/masters-programmes /master-of-public-health/
King's College London	MPH	Yes	Yes		http://www.kcl.ac.uk/study/postgraduate /taught-courses/public-health-mph-msc -mph-primary-care.aspx
University of Liverpool	MPH	No	Yes		https://www.imperial.ac.uk/medicine /study/postgraduate/masters-programmes /master-of-public-health/
Liverpool John Moores University	MSc in public health	Yes	Yes		https://www.ljmu.ac.uk/study/courses /postgraduates/public-health
London Metropolitan University	MSc in public health	Yes	Yes		http://www.londonmet.ac.uk/courses /postgraduate/public-health—msc/

(Continued)

Table 6.3 (Continued)   General UK MPH programmes

Institution	Degree awarded	Optional modules	Dissertation	Explicitly allow intercalating students?	Website
London School of Hygiene and Topical Medicine	MSc in public health	Yes	Yes	Yes	http://www.lshtm.ac.uk/study/masters/msph.html
Newcastle University	MPH	Yes	Yes	Yes	http://www.ncl.ac.uk/postgraduate/courses/degrees/public-health-mph-pgdip/
Northumbria University	MPH	No	Yes		https://www.northumbria.ac.uk/study-at-northumbria/courses/master-of-public-health-dtfpuh6/
University of Nottingham	MPH	Yes	Yes		https://www.nottingham.ac.uk/pgstudy/courses/medicine/medical-sciences/master-of-public-health-mph.aspx
Nottingham Trent University	MA in public health	Yes	Yes or research project and practical public health experience		https://www.ntu.ac.uk/study-and-courses/courses/find-your-course
Oxford Brookes University	MSc in public health	No	Yes		https://www.brookes.ac.uk/courses/postgraduate/public-health/
Queens University Belfast	MPH	Yes	Yes		http://www.qub.ac.uk/Study/Course-Finder/

(Continued)

Table 6.3 (Continued) General UK MPH programmes

Institution	Degree awarded	Optional modules	Dissertation	Explicitly allow intercalating students?	Website
University of Salford	MSc in public health	Yes	Yes		http://www.salford.ac.uk/pgt-courses/public-health
University of Sheffield	MPH	Yes	Yes	Yes	https://www.shef.ac.uk/scharr/prospective_students/masters/mph
Sheffield Hallam University	MSc in public health	Yes	Yes		https://www.shu.ac.uk/study-here/find-a-course/msc-public-health
University of Southampton	MSc in public health	Yes	Yes		http://www.southampton.ac.uk/medicine/postgraduate/taught_courses/msc_public_health_pathways.page
University of Sunderland	MSc in public health	No	No		http://www.sunderland.ac.uk/courses/appliedsciences/postgraduate/public-health/
University of Warwick	MPH	Yes	No		http://www2.warwick.ac.uk/fac/med/study/cpd/phealth/b902/
University of Wolverhampton	MPH	No	Yes		http://courses.wlv.ac.uk/course.asp?code=HL002P31UVD
University of Worcester	MSc in public health	Yes	Yes		http://www.worcester.ac.uk/courses/public-health-msc.html
University of York	MPH	Yes	Yes	Yes	http://www.york.ac.uk/healthsciences/gradschool/public-health/

Note: Table details are correct as of 2016.

MBA

Kyle Ragins with Shiv Gaglani

Why an MBA?

An MBA offers a formal education in organisational leadership. It is a degree available to medical students of certain countries, namely, the United States. As discussed elsewhere in this book, many physicians serve as organisational leaders without much or any formal education beyond medical school. Without a formal education in how to lead an organisation, many physician leaders are left with significant holes in knowledge. While not globally accessible, the last decade in the United States has seen the MBA become one of the fastest growing add-on degrees for medical students [1]. With this in mind, this chapter will focus on an MBA in medical training by drawing on the US experience.

What to expect

The MBA degree is diverse and versatile, different programmes will provide different educational opportunities. However, all programmes are geared towards providing a formal education in being an organisational leader. Typical MBA curricula are structured around a set of classes each focussed on a different functional department that most organisations will have including human relations, innovation/research and development, competitive strategy, corporate finance/accounting, operations and marketing/public relations. See the 'Management, business and leadership in medicine' section in Chapter 7 for further details on core business topics. Additionally, many MBA programmes have soft skill leadership curricula that run alongside functional classes, educating students on effective communication, motivational strategies, feedback; facilitating teamwork; and developing credibility as a leader.

Most MBA courses are structured around business cases. These challenge students to think about how organisational leaders can and should face such problems. As a medical student or junior doctor, unless this is your second career, much of the standard MBA curriculum will be new to you, and there will be a lot to learn. By the end, you will speak the language of business and know how to communicate as a leader. Of course, there will be plenty of fun extracurricular activities and time to get to know people in your programme and build your network as well.

Types of MBA programmes

There are thousands of MBA programmes across the world with different structures, curricula and focuses. Broadly speaking, there are three main types of programmes:

1. *Full-time MBA programmes* – Where students study without working for 1 or 2 years (depending on the programme and country).
2. *Part-time MBA programmes* – Where students who are working full time take classes at night or on the weekends (these programmes vary in length depending on course load).
3. *Online MBA programmes* – Where students take classes online (again varying in length depending on course load).

Some MBA programmes have specific industry focuses, e.g. a healthcare management MBA or a finance MBA. While it might seem ideal for a medical student to join a healthcare-focussed MBA programme, this can detract value from an MBA education. As most medical students spend their entire lives in the healthcare industry, being involved with people outside healthcare can expose you to different ways of thinking and approaches to problem-solving.

Organising an MBA as a medical trainee

Historically, most physicians with MBAs have done their MBAs after medical school. Once they reach leadership positions in organisations and they realise they lack a formal education in organisational leadership, they figure out some way to do an MBA. For many, this means enrolling in a part-time or online MBA programme, but some have also taken years off as mid-career professionals to pursue a full-time MBA. Now that MBA degrees are becoming more popular among physicians, the decision about when to pursue your degree is one that you can, and should, think about early in your medical career.

Before medical school

Very few medical students will pursue an MBA before medical school, in part, because in most countries medical school is an undergraduate course for students. The main linear option towards completing an MBA degree prior to medical school would be completing a combined bachelor's degree and MBA programme as an undergraduate, before entering a postgraduate medical school programme.

At medical school

The most straightforward way to achieve this is by enrolling in a combined educational programme that includes both a medical degree and an MBA. However, to date these are largely confined to North America. If these are not available, pursuing an MBA during medical school will typically require you getting permission from your medical school.

Look carefully at your medical school curriculum and figure out the most logical time to take a break from medical school to pursue the MBA. If there is a precedent of completing PhDs or MPHs while in medical school in the past, following the lead of when these students pursued their alternative studies is likely your best option. Do your research and approach your school dean/administration with a clear story about why you want to do the degree and data showing how many other universities are now facilitating this. With excellent preparation and a bit of luck, you will be well on your way to putting together your MBA-combined programme so that other students can follow in your footsteps!

After medical school

The main difficulty here is that, in many countries, it is traditional to complete a postgraduate medical training programme, or residency, in a specific clinical specialty after graduation from medical school. Taking time off during this to pursue an MBA may interrupt your timeline and could possibly make it more difficult to get into the training programme of your choice. Undertaking an MBA after specialty training might be more feasible. However, by this stage you may have many other work and personal responsibilities, making pursuing an MBA logistically too difficult.

Where to do one

It is widely accepted that the top business schools in the world are full-time, 2-year programmes in the United States. Harvard, Stanford and Wharton (at the University of Pennsylvania) are perennially considered the top three. As a medical student with excellent credentials, gaining access to one of these programmes is not out of your reach by any stretch. Every year Harvard and Stanford enrol numerous visiting medical students in their MBA programme. Duke (Fuqua) and the Yale School of Management (where I did my MBA) are also extremely welcoming to visiting medical students from other universities. There are also many 1-year programmes in Europe (and a few in North America) that are very highly regarded including London Business

School, Institut Européen d'Administration des Affaires, Cambridge (Judge School), IESE, and Oxford (Saïd School) among others. These may be better options if you are looking to limit your time away from medicine to a single year. There are numerous MBA rankings and books discussing the advantages and disadvantages of each programme. *The Financial Times* runs an annual global MBA ranking [2].

MBA vs. MPH?

I am clearly biased in answering this question, but it commonly comes up. Both the MBA and the MPH degree appeal to those who want to go beyond a single-patient encounter to improve healthcare systems and the health of a population. However, the content of the two degrees differs substantially. An MPH is largely rooted in the healthcare sector and focusses on learning information related to how healthcare is delivered, what determines the health of populations and how you might influence this. It is also devoted to developing functional quantitative skills related to epidemiology and biostatics, depending on what focus you choose to pursue with your MPH. If you are interested in being able to run statistical analyses for clinical trials or to plan and carry out medical-related research, the MPH degree will give you much more knowledge in that space than the MBA.

The MBA degree is not traditionally tied to any sector or industry. It is more focussed on learning about how to conceptualise problems faced by organisational leaders across a wide array of sectors and expose you to methods for developing successful solutions. You will learn more core business topics such as finance, accounting and marketing and much less statistics, epidemiology and econometrics (although many business schools offer advanced electives on these topics). You will also likely have more emphasis on developing your soft skills as a leader in business school than most MPH programmes offer.

Anecdote: Opening doors

After completing my combined MD–MBA programme at Yale, I found myself facing a choice between taking a job offer at a top management consulting firm versus continuing my clinical training in an emergency medicine residency programme. I felt that if I took the consulting job, I would have a hard time getting back into clinical medicine later. If I passed up the competitive consulting job,

I might have a hard time getting a similar opportunity in the future. My experience taught me that one of the most attractive parts of an MBA programme is opening doors to the recruiting process into competitive business jobs. By completing your MBA at a time other than after all your clinical training is complete, you may limit your ability to capitalise on that part of the MBA degree experience.

Case study: Founding Osmosis

Shiv Gaglani

I switched from an MD–PhD to an MD–MBA trajectory because I realised that what I enjoyed about medical research was the potential to have a broader scale impact. It was with this lens that my colleague at Johns Hopkins School of Medicine and I began working on what would become Osmosis (https://www.osmosis.org), a learning platform used by more than 50,000 medical students and officially adopted by 25 medical schools. I took a hiatus from Hopkins to pursue Osmosis and develop skills and connections through a tech incubator (DreamIt Health) and then my MBA at Harvard Business School. These experiences have made it clear that I enjoy developing scalable solutions at the intersection of healthcare and education. My advice for students interested in an MBA is to introspect and figure out what they are most passionate about – in my case, it was the ability to scale my individual work with patients and students and find ways to dissociate my time from my potential impact. It is also important to consider how your field will change in 5, 10 and 15 years so you can anticipate how your chosen profession and its role may evolve.

Conclusion

An MBA offers medical students and junior doctors an immersive and unique perspective on business, problem-solving and leadership. With it, you can do almost anything. The skills and knowledge you acquire are readily transferrable to a clinical career. And no degree will offer you the same ballast to step outside of medicine or healthcare altogether, be it in industry, start-ups or elsewhere. Best of luck!

References

1. Goyal, R., Aung, K. K., Oh, B., Hwang, T. J., Besancon, E., and Jain, S. H. AM last page: Survey of MD/MBA programmes: Opportunities for physician management education. *Acad Med: J Assoc Am Med Coll.* 2015;90(1):121.

2. *The Financial Times Ltd.* Global MBA ranking 2016. http://rankings.ft.com/businessschoolrankings/global-mba-ranking-2016. Accessed on June 14, 2017.

Further reading

Forbes. The Best Business Schools. http://www.forbes.com/business-schools/.

Poets and Quants. http://www.poetsandquants.com.

The Economist. Full time MBA ranking. http://www.economist.com/whichmba /full-time-mba-ranking.

US News. 2018 Best Business Schools. http://grad-schools.usnews.rankings andreviews.com/best-graduate-schools/top-business-schools.

NON-DEGREE STUDENT

Ashton Barnett-Vanes

Background: No degree?

To some (your parents?), this might seem like a non-starter, but there are plenty of advantages to taking out a period to conduct specialist study or research – even when it will not lead to the awarding of a degree. These opportunities have a number of names: 'visiting scholar', 'special student' and so on, but the main concept is the same. These opportunities are often taken by medical students or junior doctors who are keen to develop skills or experience in a diverse range of fields allied to or outside of medicine. Non-degree opportunities are designed to offer a great deal of flexibility to students. You might wish to partake in a semester of activity or a whole year, a decision which may be made for you if you are applying for a scholarship. This chapter will highlight these comparably lesser-known opportunities and provide information to guide your approach.

Choosing where to go

Non-degree studies are offered by universities and institutions for a number of reasons. For the institute, it enables them to attract talent to engage in its activities on a more flexible basis and without the need to award them all degrees. For students, it offers you the chance to build your own programme of courses or research activity which suits your interests and timescale. Many universities, particularly the top institutes from across the world, offer visiting or exchange programmes for students including those in the United Kingdom, the United States, Singapore, China and many more.

In deciding where to go, you should consider the following factors:

- Does the institution offer programmes or courses that you are interested in?
- Do you have informal or formal connections to the institution or their academics?
- Is the country of study (if different from your own) suitable – can you speak the language?
- Is your plan feasible and deliverable?
- What support, financial or otherwise, is available to you?

In answering these questions, you will have prepared the basis for an application. The most important factor in this decision is *what* you want to do and not necessarily *where* you are doing it. As you get no formal degree at the end, you will need to reap the most from the opportunities offered to justify it to yourself and, more importantly, your medical school course/programme director. There are drawbacks to this: you are not guaranteed anything apart from some course credits, which may not be useful for your medical qualification; you will disrupt your medical training and be out of sync with your year group; and you are likely to incur financial costs associated with relocation and eventual return. Still interested? I knew you would be, read on. . . .

Making an application

Applying to be a non-degree student is going to require some logistical planning. You will need to interrupt your studies at medical school and coordinate your application accordingly. You may be able to get financial support for this, either from your university or by applying for scholarships. In the United Kingdom, prestigious scholarships include those offered by the Kennedy Memorial Trust, Fullbright Commission and British Council. Although their provisions vary, most scholarships will include a stipend and the covering of tuition fees. Some will also help facilitate academic connections or project development ahead of your arrival.

To apply, you will need a personal statement; academic references; and other supporting material such as a study plan or project proposal, CV and so on. Again, deadlines will be months if not years ahead of departure, so plan well in advance. While not essential, some form of connection with the country or institution you are going to may help your application. If you have already visited there as a tourist, or performed work with their academics – these details could be influential in demonstrating the prior thought and planning that underpins your latest endeavour.

Arriving and succeeding

If you are successful in your application – congratulations! Arriving at a new institution will be exciting, but it is natural to feel anxious or lost at the beginning. The first step to settling in is to get accustomed to your new environment. Go on an introductory tour at your new university if there is one. There might be induction schemes for new students, even specific ones for non-degree visiting students, as you are likely to be one of hundreds if not thousands of other visitors. If you are taking a range of classes or courses, you will need to familiarise yourself with the landscape of the campus or city and the required course material. You may be required or have the option to sit exams. Sitting the exams will ensure you learn the content but will bring on the usual stress of revision and might constrain your freedom at a time when there is much else to be gained. Should you not wish to do exams but still sit in the course lectures and tutorials, this is called 'auditing'. If you are participating in research, meet your supervisors and department quickly and develop/finalise your project. In some ways, the fixed shorter timeline you have (one semester or one year) helps to kick things off at a high tempo.

Either way, the fact that you are not a degree student gives you the freedom to roam widely. Visiting students are often high-calibre with a penchant for networking; this experience could therefore serve as a great opportunity to build your professional and personal network and establish new friendships and collaborations. While the amount you can achieve in a semester or year is limited, non-degree visits give you the chance to impress future colleagues or supervisors. For example, if you are passionate about public health but do not have the CV to apply for a PhD yet, a non-degree year could be a good opportunity to build face time and rapport with top academics from other institutions in the field. Here, the non-degree project serves as a stepping stone towards a future major opportunity. If you do manage to publish or present work performed during your visit, share it with your medical school and sponsor if applicable; this helps build 'guanxi'* all round.

Leaving

While it is important to make a good entrance, leaving is also an art worth perfecting. Get your supervisors and key colleagues a small gift or card and offer to keep in touch every 6 months. Many students come

---

* A Chinese term for the cultivation of influential networks and relationships, written as 关系.

and go, but most do not maintain relationships down the line. These are what you will want to leverage should you one day decide you are ready to apply for that PhD.

Conclusion

Non-degree study is as good as you make it. If you have a longer-term plan to establish yourself in a given field or compete for a higher-degree or position at an institution, a non-degree can be a powerful vehicle in support of this aim. However, the greater flexibility that comes with these opportunities means you must have high levels of self-drive and discipline. While the time and cost implications are not insignificant, scholarship or sponsorship can offset most if not all these with proper planning. Picking your own courses and building your own research project is a unique experience – enjoy it!

Further reading

There are a huge number of visiting student options around the world, each with their own forms of funding and scholarship. Notable and highly competitive ones include the following:

British Council. https://www.britishcouncil.org/.

Fulbright Commission. http://www.fulbright.org.uk/.

Kennedy Scholarship. http://www.kennedytrust.org.uk.

Pros

- Highly flexible programme that can be tailored to your interests
- International experience often with top academics and institutions
- Chance to compete for prestigious scholarships and build a network of contacts from around the world

Cons

- Highly competitive and require significant advanced planning
- Disrupts your medical training
- Can be a costly exercise for few immediate tangible gains

CHAPTER 7

Design, innovation and management

CONTENTS

DESIGN AND INNOVATION IN MEDICINE

Maniragav Manimaran with Neomi Bennett

Background

Medicine and healthcare is an ever-changing field. Innovating in medicine can yield incredible outcomes, but the development process is both complex and time consuming. Often, a first-hand clinical experience is necessary to understand a health problem and develop a viable solution. Medical and healthcare students have an ideal vantage point to contribute towards – or even lead – impactful innovations in healthcare: they have an extensive scientific background, invaluable clinical experience and comparatively more time to pursue new ideas.

From problem to idea

Find the problem

The first step is to spot a problem that bothers you, something you are passionate about. It is essential that the problem motivates you, as there is little else that will help propel you at the outset of a project. Think back to when you have been frustrated in a healthcare placement:

- Were patients waiting unnecessarily?
- Did it take too long to get key test results on the online system?
- Could the medical procedure you observed be done more efficiently?

Once you have observed a problem, it is important to understand whether there is a need for a solution. In other words, your peers, patients and/or medical colleagues need to agree that it is a problem too. If they do not – can you persuade them? If not, you are unlikely to develop a viable solution with clinical impact. This highlights the importance of getting feedback early from relevant stakeholders.

Brainstorming ideas

Once you have identified a problem, it is time to develop a list of viable solutions. Your first solution is almost never the best, so you should be open to pivoting and evolving your idea as you gain feedback. Do not let the fear of someone stealing your idea stop you from doing effective market research (see intellectual property [IP] considerations later), as the benefit of gaining valuable advice from stakeholders can often outweigh the risks.

Market research and estimation

Thorough market research is vital for assessing competitors/market size in the early stages of innovation. You need to become familiar with not only the problem, but also its implications, current work-arounds and patient/provider perspectives. As a medical student, you are expected to shadow clinicians, and this can afford you cutting-edge insight; even if you have to do this outside of your normal timetable, it is worth the effort. When approaching clinicians, be specific about why you want to shadow them as they can help tailor cases relevant to your needs. Do not be disheartened if they take a long time to respond (or do not respond).

Having identified a viable solution, it is important that you estimate the potential market size that you are targeting. At first glance, this can seem very daunting – how on earth are you supposed to know how many people will use your product? The key is that you should break everything down to first principles. Equip yourself with some key statistics, searching on your local health authority's website or the WHO's can often prove invaluable. Box 7.1 has some key questions to get you started.

Box 7.1   Determining your market

1. Does your problem primarily affect patients, healthcare providers or both?
2. Is your problem related to a common or rare medical/healthcare issue?
3. Does the prevalence vary depending on population ethnicities or geography?
4. How many people are affected by the problem each week in your local hospital?
   - You can extrapolate to find the estimated annual incidence in your hospital/regionally and/or use national statistics.
   - Continue this method to encompass other countries or look for a global registry to make a global estimate.

Building the right team

Once you have developed an innovation for a problem, received positive feedback from key stakeholders and have been able demonstrate that there is indeed a market – you are ready to make your innovation happen. For this, you will need a great team around you. When you arc in the early stages of your product development, it is best to think of your idea as a project rather than a start-up. This simple thought process allows you to focus more on building a good product rather than excessively on financials; you can transition to a start-up once you have registered your company.

You may already have a partner or co-founder for your idea. However, it is common that as your project evolves, you may need new people with unique skill sets in order to advance to the next stage. In entrepreneurship, the classical founding team is often thought to consist of a *hacker*, a *hustler/visionary* and a *designer*. The hacker is the technological maverick in the team, the go-to person with extensive knowledge of the functionality and inner workings of the product. The hustler/visionary is a person who drives the team forward, manages the project and has a vision for the end product. The designer is someone who understands what the market wants and helps shape the product to positively enhance brand identity/penetration.

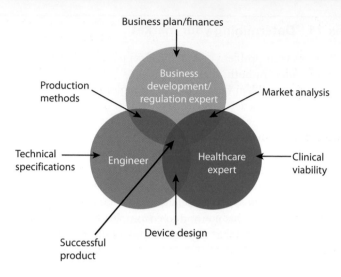

Figure 7.1 Medical innovation team.

These categories are just an outline and by no means does your team need to have people to fit all (or any) these. But what it does show is the importance of having a group of people with a diverse and complementary set of skills to navigate the complexities of medical innovation. Figure 7.1 illustrates an example team designing a medical device and how their roles combine to develop a successful product.

Product development and intellectual property

Prototyping

It is best to try and get a working prototype of your device/app as soon as possible (within the first few months of developing your medical innovation). This is because, as you actively develop and build the idea, you will start to understand the complexities and practicalities of your solution beyond what is possible at the design stage.

For example, for medical device innovation, this can be done by using computer-aided design (CAD) software such as FreeCAD, Blender or Sketchup. Other software, such as Meshmixer, is good for editing your prototype designs so that they can be effectively three-dimensionally (3D) printed. Moreover, Netfabb is a great software for automatically fixing your CADs so that the 3D mesh is free from errors and can be suitably printed. If you are creating mobile applications or web software, there are many tools that you can use even if you are not familiar with coding. For example, you can use online tools such as InVision to create a simple shell of your application, Wix to create a simple website and GitHub to manage your project across your team. Developing a prototype early on will allow you to pivot and evolve your idea sooner, accelerating your progress in the long term.

IP

IP encompasses any product of the human mind that has market value and includes a range of considerations including copyrights, trademarks and patents. It is vital that you pay attention to this early on in your project. The most commonly discussed IP consideration is patents, a legal document that gives an individual exclusive commercial rights over their invention for a specified time period. This prevents other people from using your idea while your patent is valid. Patents may not be required in all cases, and each individual situation is unique. Therefore, it is important to enlist the support from an expert in IP law to identify exactly what you need in order to protect your medical innovation.

As a medical student, filing for a patent can be an expensive, complex and unfamiliar process. Therefore, it is advisable to utilise resources of your university and maximise the support available to you. Many universities have departments that support technology spin-off companies, and they can also help students to navigate the process of protecting their IP. Do note that if your medical innovation is a spin-off project from research carried out at your university, you may be required to share (or entirely give away) IP rights to your university. Again, this is highly dependent on your own situation, and so it is imperative that you seek the best possible advice from your mentors and local IP departments. Be cautious in how you approach negotiations – ideas or projects with considerable impact or earning potential will focus minds, and it is important that you are well advised prior to formally signing or agreeing to anything.

Funding, pitching and bringing to market
Advantages of lean product development
When establishing medical innovations as a medical student, it is useful to build your product lean (spending as little money as possible) by utilising your university resources. This has numerous benefits, not least by demonstrating your motivation, resourcefulness and efficiency to investors; further, you can easily pivot and change your idea without being bound by contracts and weighty expectations.

Table 7.1   Common sources of idea/start-up funding

Sources of funding	Link
Kickstarter (crowdfunding)	https://www.kickstarter.com
Crowdcube (crowdfunding)	https://www.crowdcube.com
Seedrs (crowdfunding)	https://www.seedrs.com
UCLU entrepreneurs (UCL – equity-free funding)	http://ucle.co/TheFund
Kickstart London (pre-accelerator)	http://www.kickstartldn.co.uk
Entrepreneur handbook (UK start-up competitions)	http://entrepreneurhandbook.co.uk/competitions-award/
Mass challenge (accelerator)	http://masschallenge.org

When you examine the business model of early stage start-ups, you will realise that you do not often need significant funding (if any) to begin the process of growing. Search out university-based or affiliated business advisors, look out for start-up funding competitions and take advantage of free university workspace. These all help build your product with minimal capital requirements. Once you have identified exactly how much funding you need (and what you need it for), I would recommend that you look for innovation grants/competitions, accelerator programmes or crowdfunding sources (see Table 7.1 for examples). Just be wary of whether there are any conditions for the funding that you receive (e.g. do you have to pay it back or give away any ownership of your company?). Further, find a mentor(s) to guide your innovation journey and offer insight into key business decisions. As discussed earlier, draw on a diversity of mentors from different aspects of your product/idea, e.g. entrepreneurs, clinicians, patients.

Investors and equity

Once you have bootstrapped your idea as much as you can, there will come a point when you will need to obtain funding to take your concept further. This is when you should start reaching out to investors. A key consideration in the early stages of your innovation journey is to understand how much equity (ownership of your company), if any, you are willing to give in exchange for funding. Giving away significant amounts of equity is something to be careful about. It is worth discussing with your team or mentor from the outset. From an investor's viewpoint, investing in early-stage ideas is a risky business because many ideas are not profitable, hence why investors want to get a high equity share. From a founder's viewpoint, giving away too much equity may dilute your ownership/control over the company. On the other hand, without sufficient funding, you may not have the necessary resources to bring your idea to market. These viewpoints outline the complexities when searching for funding, and it is important to make sure that you have done a thorough risk–benefit analysis.

Angel investors are individuals who provide funding or capital for early stage companies in exchange for some ownership equity. Venture capital investments are usually from a group of investors or a pooled fund which is used to invest in a start-up in exchange for equity. As a generalisation, angel investors may be more suitable for early-stage seed rounds (for example, £5,000–£200,000), and venture capital investments are often for larger investment rounds once you have proven the viability of your business (often £100,000–£1 million).

Anecdote: University funders

As president of the University College London Union (UCLU) Entrepreneurs Society in 2015/2016, I helped secure a record £12,000 in funding to support our society events and our venture capital fund. Consequently, I helped invest over £7000 in student businesses at UCL. The best start-ups that we funded were those who had identified a tangible objective and presented a clear plan to achieve it.

Approaching investors

When reaching out to investors, cold calls or e-mails often do not have a high success rate. The best way for you to get onto their radar is to find someone to personally introduce you. This can seem daunting but that is what networking is for. Attend a variety of events related to your field, make connections and follow them up using LinkedIn. Once you have caught an investor's attention, you will need to make a formal business plan/pitch deck, presentation or both.

Pitching your idea

Business plans and pitch decks (a brief set of slides used to present your business) are dependent on your individual needs and the type of product you are developing. Although there are some classical structures for business plans, there is no one-size-fits-all formula because every product is different (or should be). As a guideline, Box 7.2 has some key factors to address; see Chapter 4 for details on presenting.

Box 7.2   What to include in a pitch

1. *Concept* – How much potential is there behind your idea or service? Is it original?
2. *Development* – What is your current development stage? How much effort have you put in?
3. *Market potential* – Have you proven a market demand for your idea? How much of a gap is there in the market?
4. *Financials* – What is your projected growth/expected revenue? How do you hope to monetise your product? What are your profit margins?
5. *Product feasibility* – How realistic is your design in terms of cost, technical requirements and timescale to develop?
6. *Competitive differentiation* – How unique is your product/ service compared to the rest of the competitors in the market? How will you make your idea stand out?
7. *Branding* – How appealing is your brand name and logo? Will it attract customers?
8. *Why you?* – This is perhaps the most important factor to address. Investors are investing in you as much as they are investing in your idea, and so you have to show them your own original way of thinking and highlight why they should take a risk and invest in you.

Once investors are happy with your proposal, they will do their own due diligence to check the feasibility of your idea, financial projections and validity of your market predictions. Once satisfied, they will make a proposal for funding in exchange for equity.

Taking to market

The process of taking your idea to market does not usually happen in one step. For example, in the case of apps, once it has been alpha-tested internally by the developing team, it is often released to a select group of external users for beta testing before it is released to the public. When launching, it is important to find early adopters who would be willing to try your product, help you test it and share it across their network to give you more market momentum. Once your product is ready, you will need to establish an effective marketing campaign targeted at the right audience prior to launch. This will help build the excitement and anticipation before you release your product, thus leading to maximum impact at launch.

Case study: Neo-slip

Neomi Bennett

As a student nurse at Kingston University in London, the research I conducted highlighted that 25,000 patients die each year of deep vein thrombosis (DVT); anti-embolism stockings are used to prevent this condition in postoperative patients. I noticed that many people (especially the elderly) had difficulty applying anti-embolism stockings due to their tightness, leading to reduced patient use. This is how the idea for Neo-slip arose. I wrote about the concept in an essay which caught the attention of teachers and went on to carry out experiments with various materials to create a simple to use garment that enables patients to slide stockings over it. The aim of Neo-slip was to promote increased usage of anti-embolism stockings by making their application easier and quicker, which in turn can significantly reduce loss of life through DVTs.

Once I had a prototype, I put together focus groups with patients, nurses and doctors. I worked with university graduates to help develop and design packaging and was contacted by the NHS after catching their attention on social media. I then collaborated with the NHS to gain a better understanding of their requirements and quality standards. Having studied nursing, I have had to learn about business structures and processes in my own time while taking the product to market. Neo-slip is now CE marked signifying its compliance with the relevant EU directives regarding health and safety.

There were financial challenges to overcome, as cash flow is vital for the success of a start-up company. I joined business networking groups, which enabled me to learn the foundations of business. In addition, I took advantage of a government start-up loan, and this included a mentor, which was extremely useful in the start-up phase of the business. Neo-slip recently became available on NHS prescription (FP10), meaning older patients (the most vulnerable) can now receive Neo-slip free of charge from their general practitioner. My innovation has improved patient care and taken me on a whirlwind journey, including meeting the UK Prime Minister at No 10 Downing Street.

My top tips are as follows:

1. Hire the right people to do the work.
2. Test your market.
3. Build a positive network to support you.
4. Do not think too long, just take action.
5. Enjoy the journey and remember to look after yourself.

Good luck!

Conclusion

Innovating in medicine is hard work, but it is also an extremely exciting process! Building an awesome team around your idea makes all the difference and will allow you to create great solutions that solve relevant problems. Medical innovators can make a lasting mark on the healthcare industry – now it is your turn to seize the opportunity!

Common pitfalls

1. *Insufficient market research.*

    It is important to establish a valid need for your product before developing the solution; contact as many clinicians, patients and key stakeholders as you can. The process may take a few weeks or months, but it is important that you invest the time in the early stages of your project to avoid problems later.

2. *Having an ineffective team.*

    Sometimes, your team may not have all the skills needed to develop your product. Occasionally, some members of your team could become demotivated, and their lack of involvement can bring down the rest of your project. It is important to realise this early so that you can actively make the changes to ensure that your team has the skill set required to build your innovation.

3. *Limited market potential.*

    You need to ensure that your innovation has a sufficiently large potential market so that your idea can be scaled up in the long term. Moreover, investors often expect a minimum future market potential; hence, without a sufficiently large market, you may struggle to get appropriate funding. Make sure that you have clear reasoning behind your estimated market size as this is a key factor with regard to investor funding decisions.

Further reading

Product design:

Blender. https://www.blender.org.

FreeCad. http://www.freecadweb.org.

Meshmixer. http://www.meshmixer.com.

Netfabb. https://www.netfabb.com.

SketchUp. http://www.sketchup.com.

App/website development:

Github. https://github.com.

Invision. https://www.invisionapp.com/#.

Wix. http://www.wix.com.

Useful links:

Biodesign. http://ebiodesign.org.

BMJ Innovations. http://innovations.bmj.com.

Kickstart London. http://www.kickstartldn.co.uk.

Neo-slip. http://neo-slip.co.uk/.

MANAGEMENT, BUSINESS AND LEADERSHIP IN MEDICINE

Edgar Meyer

Introduction

In the United Kingdom, recent years have seen the NHS struggle on many fronts. For example, we know that the financial pressures on the healthcare systems are immense. Consider the changing demographics, the increased pressure of managing a fair and accessible system for all at a time when working patterns and expectations are changing or the growing demands placed on healthcare to deal with long-term conditions and multiple co-morbidities. Issues such as these are, however, not unique to the United Kingdom, and you will find healthcare systems in other countries, both developed and developing, facing similar challenges. Yet strikingly, in the face of these and other challenges, medical curricula remain largely devoid of any formal education on management, business acumen or leadership. This is even more perplexing if one considers that progression through specialist training pathways in the United Kingdom is reliant on you demonstrating management and leadership skills/potential.

> Often as a medical student you inadvertently limit yourself to the skills that medical school has to offer and fail to realise your true potential because you are so focused on just becoming a doctor. However, doing management helped me to realise that I have so much more to

offer. Not only has it embellished me as a developing clinician through improved leadership and management skills, but it has given me the confidence to see myself as more than just a medic. (Elisabeth Simisola Oke, 2016)

Why study business/management?

There is now growing consensus for the need to engage doctors in the leadership and management of the NHS, with proponents emphasising the importance of clinical leaders, in particular doctors, to ensure sustainable quality of service. Indeed, research suggests that doctors in training are seeking further development and, at present, are an underutilised and underdeveloped resource that could contribute significantly to the development of the NHS [1]. Studying supplementary programmes in business-, management- and/or leadership-related subjects will not make you a perfect manager or leader in healthcare. However, what such courses can deliver is the opportunity for you to understand business principles, develop different perspectives, hone your teamwork and leadership abilities and consider solutions to dynamic problems facing healthcare now and going forward. Having delivered business and management programmes to medics for many years, the feedback is generally supportive of such an assumption.

The management degree has already allowed me to better engage in service improvement, audit and research. . . . [It] has allowed me to understand the context in which I work in, allowing me to develop towards my career aspirations. (Meelad Sayma, 2016)

What will you learn?

You need to consider carefully what you want to gain from a programme that focusses on business-related content. Many of you may be worried to leave medicine for a period – contemplating how this may impact your opportunities to progress as a medic. Anecdotal evidence suggests that the experience of being part of a different environment not only outweighs any potential drawbacks, but can also bring added advantages to students. But like with so many things, it is what you make of these opportunities. Different programmes will offer different insights, teaching approaches and opportunities. You need to decide what is important to you. No management programme will make you an expert. These programmes aim to build foundations and insights by challenging you, enabling you to ask intelligent questions. You may want to consider the following list as indicative content that would allow you to have a broad understanding of the complexities of managing in organisations, with a specific focus on managing and leading within healthcare.

- *Finance and accounting.*

    I am sure not everyone will be enthusiastic about the idea of studying such subjects. However, if you are responsible for budgets, managing complex medical technologies, or are responsible for a team of healthcare staff, you do need to understand the basics of how organisations use financial information to make decisions.

- *Strategy and business environment.*

    Irrespective of the organisation you work in – public, private or charitable – understanding the context in which you operate is pivotal. Information about the environment may include competitors, suppliers or ecological considerations of business practices. Understanding such information will enable you to devise and refine a plan of where the organisation may need to be in the future and how it must to adapt to get to a desired state. Developing such a plan and vision for the future is usually captured in business strategy. Thinking ahead and using information about your context is an essential analytical skill for any manager and leader.

- *Business functions.*

    Each programme will emphasise different aspects related to running a business. Some programmes introduce you to functions such as marketing, ensuring that you understand a range of perspectives on how to communicate messages. Organisational behaviour, human resource management and leadership are often covered – albeit in different guises. Make sure you have the opportunity to learn about these facets of management. In subjects related to these areas of business management, you look at the psychology of people, the dynamics of teams, how to motivate and incentivise people and what it means to be a leader. These are not merely soft skills, but they are ideas and models that can help you be more effective once you are responsible for people and projects in any organisation.

- *Healthcare-related subjects.*

    Some management programmes may speak to you as a medical practitioner, although there is nothing wrong with generic business and management programmes. Such healthcare-focussed programmes may cover areas that are immediately relevant to what you, as clinicians, will experience. Examples may include how to manage healthcare organisations; often, such organisations work in complex and unique environments with idiosyncratic characteristics heavily shaped by government politics. The programme should cover some economics content – health economics courses are fascinating, as they develop your ability to analytically look at relationships and efficiencies within systems. Some programmes also look at the use and management of information in healthcare. This may take the form of courses on health informatics or the way in which information is used to influence policy. Technology has become pervasive, and healthcare is no exception. You need to understand the impact technological advances have on your practice. This could be related to information sharing or the use of apps as a means to monitor or facilitate better health.

Changing the way you think

Some programmes offer modules that, on first appearance, bear no relevance to medical degrees or business management in general. Subjects such as entrepreneurship or innovation may not sound like they are necessary for you as medical students – but consider this: Entrepreneurship is not about Richard Branson or Dyson; it is about how we take an idea to market. As discussed in the previous chapter, as medics, you may develop an idea about a treatment, a medical technology or indeed a new solution to an existing problem. How are you going to make this work in practice? What resources do you need to transform your idea into a reality? These are the kind of questions courses on entrepreneurship may offer you. The same applies to innovation; this is not necessarily about developing the next model of an X-ray machine or a new inhaler for asthma sufferers (although, it could be). But rather how you engage in design thinking – developing solutions to problems is a process, and courses on innovation may support your understanding in these areas.

There is no right or wrong choice, and you will need to consider how broad you want your training to be or if you want to maintain a more tailored focus on medicine and healthcare; your decision should be guided by your motivation and desire and should speak to your career ambitions.

Where to go?

For medical students, the choices are limited in regard to formal management training as part of the curriculum – at least in the United Kingdom. There are two intercalated programmes in the United Kingdom that medical students can take as part of their BSc qualification – one at Imperial College Business School, a programme that has been established in 1997, and a programme more recently launched at King's College London. Other opportunities present themselves through summer schools or short course options. Such programmes, if provided by good and reputable institutions, are a good way to get a flavour of business and management studies.

My experience has shown me that many medical practitioners are taking time out of their specialist training to upskill themselves through MBAs (see 'The MBA' section in Chapter 6) or other master-level programmes, such as specific MSc programmes that either focus on a particular management and leadership topic or are more generic. Different countries will offer variations of such programmes, and listing all variants is nigh impossible. From experience, I have seen an increase in medics joining more traditional business and management programmes in recognition that such training is necessary to drive change for sustainable healthcare. A recent MBA graduate of mine told me that

> I have a duty to provide the best possible care to my patients, and the MBA has highlighted to me that quality of care is not limited to diagnostic acumen or surgical skill. If a department full of talented and hardworking clinicians is unable to ensure that outpatient clinics run on time, or cannot control an ever-expanding waiting list, then I believe that we as clinicians have a duty to better equip ourselves to address these issues. (Rory Nicholson, 2016)

Many deaneries have leadership and management development programmes. Most of these sit outside specialist training pathways and require you to take time out of your specialist training or attend these on top of your rotations and specialist training requirements. The opportunities depend on the deanery you are in, but could take the forms of sabbaticals, time abroad or speaker series. I am aware of exchange programmes in the United States, project-based work in developing countries or bespoke research programmes. The United States offers a number of specialist programmes for medics that focus on management in healthcare.

It is important to note that there is no right or wrong pathway! The important message is that you ought to engage with management, leadership and business ideas. The development in your thinking, the appreciation of the challenges from a different perspective and the additional tools and techniques will only make you a better clinician. Whether such programmes are focussed on healthcare directly or are more general in their approach is a decision that you have to take. One advantage of a more general management programme is the ability to network with, and learn from, people with different perspectives.

Outcomes

Many management programmes have a project component. These are prime opportunities to develop publishable materials. I know of numerous cases where dissertations or final projects have been presented at international conferences or in peer-reviewed journals. Some business and management programmes may allow you the freedom to develop ideas for products and/or services. For an example, see the 'Further reading' section. In terms of your career, understanding management, leadership and business will enable you to apply more confidently to senior managerial posts, as you can demonstrate a more insightful approach to understanding the complexities that exist within a given healthcare context.

Conclusion

Where does this leave you? There is no perfect programme nor is there an ultimate level of knowledge to be achieved that will guarantee you success. It is about development and about the willingness to engage in a different way of thinking to ensure that you can contribute to the best of your ability for the good of patients.

I would like to end with another quotation from a specialist registrar, who took time out to engage in a year-long management programme:

> As a specialty registrar, studying [management] has changed my perspective on our role within the NHS. It has demystified the processes by which the NHS is managed and governed and has enabled me to better understand the perspectives of hospital administrators. It has drawn my attention to aspects of the NHS which are unusual amongst other industries and has given me a toolkit of generic problem-solving techniques. . . . At the end of the day, we are all trying to achieve the best

possible quality of care for our patients, using a finite set of resources. This would be easier if we all spoke a common language, and I hope that a better engagement with the organisational functions of healthcare will soon become a more formalised component of medical training and practice. (Rory Nicholson, 2016)

Reference

1. Gilbert, A., Hockey, P., Vaithianathan, R., Curzen, N., and Lees, P. Perceptions of junior doctors in the NHS about their training: Results of a regional questionnaire. *BMJ Qual Saf.* 2012;21(3): 234–8.

Further reading

Nicol, E. D. Capitalising on leadership fellowships for clinicians in the NHS. *Clin Med.* 2011;11(2): 125–7.

See a final project that has received over 70 press mentions internationally for the development of a gamified smoking cessation app (http://www.quitgenius .com/).

The Kings's Fund. *The Future of Leadership and Management in the NHS: No More Heroes.* London, p. 38. 2011.

Acknowledgements

Thank you to all the medical students and doctors who shared their views and experiences in preparation for this chapter, including Elisabeth Simisola Oke, Rory Nicholson and Meelad Sayma.

CHAPTER 8

Medical law, ethics and teaching

CONTENTS

MEDICAL LAW

Andrew Papanikitas

What is law in medicine and why get involved?

A straight answer to this question can sound a little philosophical! Doctors and other clinicians are citizens of the country they live in and subject to the same laws as everyone else. However, they do things that others generally cannot do: they record confidential information and contact details of patients and perform procedures that if done by a non-clinician or for a non-therapeutic purpose would be regarded as an assault. Debates around whether to change or how to interpret the law in practice are often ethical in nature. However, the law provides working 'answers' to what is obligatory, permissible or prohibited in healthcare practice. In the United Kingdom, there are broadly two types of law: law that is enacted by the government (statutes) and law that has developed over time as cases and which are used to develop the interpretation of statutes and previous cases (case law) [1]. Professional bodies develop guidelines for practice based on key legislation or case law. Law affects professionals in two key ways: by defining their professional duties and boundaries (or anyone could claim to be a healthcare professional such as a doctor or nurse) and by establishing society's consensus on what people (including professionals) may or may not and should or should not do. The law also relies on facts; has the law been broken?

Getting involved in medical law means acquiring the tools to understand, interpret and apply the law – to avoid falling foul of it, to teach others or to make sure that others are in line with the rules enshrined by society. It may also mean developing the skills to see when the law does not work as it should and the tools with which to either change how a law works (e.g. through the courts) or develop new laws (e.g. through the government). It can also mean developing the expertise to provide the facts that courts need in order to decide whether a law has been broken – which is where forensic experts and expert witnesses are involved. The facts can be as disputed as the law. Depending on how you want to get involved, there could be a possible career in medical law or legal medicine.

Opportunities at medical school and during medical training

Medical law, like medical ethics is included in medical school curricula (for example, see the 2010 curriculum statement on medical ethics and law listed in the references at the end of this chapter). At a basic level, key concepts such as consent, capacity and confidentiality are compulsory elements threaded throughout most medical degrees around the world. In the United Kingdom and many other settings, medical students may get the opportunity to take an interest in medical law further, for example, in a self-selected component or an elective placement or project. Most universities will also have extracurricular activities, such as evening lectures that are open to university members and even the public. Some of these activities are discussed further in the following.

BSc, BA or MA in medical law and ethics

There are now several bachelor-level degrees in medical law, some of which can be taken as an intercalated degree. Both undergraduate- and postgraduate-taught degrees usually combine medical law and ethics. The usual format is to have formative (do the essay and get feedback as learning rather than assessment) as well as graded coursework essays, a dissertation of usually around 10,000 words and a timed examination. Some courses will have closed book exams, and others will allow you to take law materials to the exam. This does not make the examinations any easier! I did the MA in medical law and ethics at King's College London. Like many other such degrees, it was available full-time or part-time. My colleagues at the time included solicitors who wished to specialise in medical law, doctors involved in forensic or medical defence work and doctors and scientists who wanted to develop an academic or educational interest in medical law and ethics. I did it full time as a sabbatical, but many of my medically qualified colleagues did it part time over 2 years and worked alongside. Bear in mind that a degree in medical law carries a heavy workload in terms of reading preparation and coursework and very often will open up extracurricular opportunities. This may include opportunities to hear about legal developments from key medicolegal figures, to attend conferences and to develop interests that might turn into publications or research projects. Most if not all degrees in medical law will either interview prospective candidates or invite a personal statement with the application materials. For this reason, it is worth thinking about why you are applying. If you are considering changing career to law, rather than specialising in medical law, it may be worth considering an ordinary law degree or an intensive 1–2-year law conversion course.

Self-selected components

Medical schools that offer self-selected components (SSCs) may have opportunities to do a medicolegal project. As a fourth year medical student, I did a medical law SSC that looked at how the law was applied through the case of the conjoined twins from Gozo, Jodie and Mary (court pseudonyms) in the High Court and the Court of Appeal. The court case examined several legal arguments in considering whether it was lawful to separate the twins in the knowledge that with surgery, one twin would definitely die, but without, both would die. For a description of the case see the study by Sheldon and Wilkinson [2]. An SSC need not be so court judgement focussed. For example, there may be opportunities to do an SSC in forensic medicine or forensic pathology. There may be the option of a self-directed library project, but remember that this still requires someone to mark the resulting work, and it still requires you to come up with a worthy research question.

Electives

The elective project is for many medical schools an assessed component of the medical degree, and despite statements to the contrary, non-clinical electives are harder to justify to your medical school. Consider having a well-defined project with implications for clinical practice. If there is a clinical component that can be built in – this may go down better with the medical school. It also means that you keep your clinical skills alive for the final year or foundation doctor jobs. An elective may offer the opportunity to publish on medicolegal topics.

Anecdote: A medicolegal elective

My elective project compared the medical malpractice insurance environment in the United Kingdom with that in the United States. At the time, a large United States-based insurance company was active in both countries. The insurance company in question was supporting medical student activities (many medical defence organisations still do), so consider whether an indemnity organisation offers bursaries or scholarships for these purposes.

Future career in medical law?

In their infamous *So You Want to Be a Brain Surgeon?* careers guide, Eccles and Sanders [3] itemise the types of medicolegal careers as follows:

- Doctor who interacts with the courts (e.g. expert witness, forensic pathologist, occupational health)
- Research and teaching law applied to medicine
- Institutional roles requiring/favouring medicolegal expertise (e.g. medical management or politics)
- Law firms, regulatory bodies, medical defence organisations (e.g. medicolegal advisor, solicitor or barrister)

The job openings in law firms and medical indemnity work are often subject to much competition. Unlike medicine, where nearly all graduates are able to get a job, it is the opposite for law graduates, many of whom end up in other careers. Medicolegal advisor posts often prefer candidates who have clinical experience as a qualified doctor or other healthcare professional. Those who have completed their specialist training are in a stronger position to apply. It is worth checking whether an indemnity organisation will cover salary and the costs of a law conversion course while a successful applicant retrains. Medical law is not an easy option. Believe it or not, medicolegal advisers do their version of on-calls! This is because some situations need medicolegal advice immediately or urgently, even on evenings and weekends. Career progression in medicolegal careers is also highly competitive.

National associations and societies in the United Kingdom

The main professional association and registration body of doctors in the United Kingdom, the British Medical Association and the General Medical Council, publish extensive guidance on the legal responsibilities of doctors [4–6]. All qualified doctors in the United Kingdom are obliged to have medical indemnity. The indemnity bodies in the United Kingdom, the Medical Protection Society, the Medical Defence Union and the Medical and Dental Defence Union of Scotland, all run educational activities for students and qualified doctors and have a database of educational cases which they discuss in their publications. Box 8.1 contains details of several of these societies and other specialist groups that are worth considering joining or attending their meetings.

Box 8.1   National associations and societies in the United Kingdom and worldwide

- Medical Defence Union (https://www.themdu.com)
- Medical Protection Society (https://www.mps.org.uk)
- Medical and Dental Defence Union of Scotland (https://www.mddus.com)
- *Faculty of Forensic and Legal Medicine of the Royal College of Physicians (FFLM)* is a professional body for doctors specialising in forensic and legal medicine in the United Kingdom. They offer specialist qualifications in legal medicine. The specialty covers forensic medical practitioners (forensic physicians, forensic pathologists, sexual assault examiners, and child physical and sexual

assault examiners), medicolegal advisers and medically qualified coroners. The FFLM publishes the *Journal of Forensic and Legal Medicine*. The FFLM is based at the Royal College of Physicians. (http://fflm.ac.uk/)

- *Royal Society of Medicine Clinical Forensic and Legal Section* run an annual programme of meetings and welcome students and trainees (They have an annual student and trainee poster prize). The meetings are usually held at the Royal Society of Medicine, 1 Wimpole Street, London, UK W1G 0AE. (https://www.rsm.ac.uk/sections/sections-and -networks-list/clinical-forensic-legal-medicine-section.aspx)

- *British Medicolegal Society* run the *Medico-Legal Journal* and hold meetings on medicolegal topics. (http://mlj .sagepub.com/)

- *World Association for Medical Law* (established in 1967/1970 depending on the account) is a not-for profit organisation. It aims to encourage the study and discussion of problems concerning health law, legal medicine and ethics and advancement of human rights.

Conclusion

The law is an unavoidable part of healthcare practice – there are many ways to get involved, from practicing it to policing it. The law can offer a career in medicine (legal medicine) or an alternative career to medicine (medical law). Both can be professionally rewarding but will require forward planning and plenty of work.

References

1. Garside, J. P. *Law for Doctors: Principles and Practicalities*, 3rd Edition. CRC Press, London, 2006.

2. Sheldon, S., and Wilkinson, S. On the sharpest horns of dilemma: Re A (conjoined twins). *Med Law Rev.* 2001;9:201–207.

3. Eccles, S., and Sanders, S. (eds.). *So You Want to Be a Brain Surgeon?*, 3rd Edition. Oxford University Press, Oxford, 2009.

4. English, V. et al. *Medical Ethics Today: The BMA's Handbook of Ethics and Law*, 3rd Edition. BMJ Books, London, 2012 (ebook available free

for BMA members: https://www.bma.org.uk/advice/employment/ethics /medical-ethics-today).

5. General Medical Council. http://www.gmc-uk.org/. Accessed on June 14, 2017.

6. British Medical Association. See http://www.bma.org.uk. Accessed on June 14, 2017.

Further reading

Here are examples of publications that I and one of the colleagues mentioned earlier respectively linked to our electives. (Both examples are from the United States, but you might want to consider whether other countries or other historical events are worth writing about.)

Jones, R. New York, 11 September and after. *J R Soc Med*. 2001;94:648. [A medical student's account of a forensic pathology elective in New York during the September 11th World Trade Centre attack.]

Papanikitas, A. Predatory crusaders. *Student BMJ*. 2001;09:399–442. [An article about why people in the United States suc nursing homes, written after attending a seminar while on a medicolegal elective.]

Stirrat, G. M., Johnston, C., Gillon, R., and Boyd, K. Medical ethics and law for doctors of tomorrow: The 1998 consensus statement updated. *J Med Ethics*. 2010;36:55–60.

MEDICAL ETHICS

Sophia Haywood and Jasmin Lovestone

What is ethics in medicine?

Medical ethics is a branch of philosophy that provides the moral framework through which we make medical decisions about patient treatment and interaction with colleagues and how we consider ourselves as doctors. It is how we ask ourselves whether we are doing the right thing for our patients – both on the individual case level and considering the impact on wider society. Sometimes more than one option may be indicated in the management of a patient. When this happens, using medical ethics can help decide which is the most moral and appropriate.

Core themes and topics

Four principles approach

Medical ethics is usually about the consideration of four principles: autonomy, beneficence, non-maleficence and justice. In different circumstances, different principles take precedence depending on the issue at stake. See Figure 8.1.

Key topics to consider

- *Consent and capacity*

    Patient's ability to make decisions for themselves

- *Confidentiality*

    Keeping patient details private

- *End-of-life decisions*

    Many tricky scenarios at the end of life – including do not resuscitate orders, assisted dying and withdrawal of care

- *Resource allocation*

    How to decide where the money is spent and how much time and effort to spend on each patient

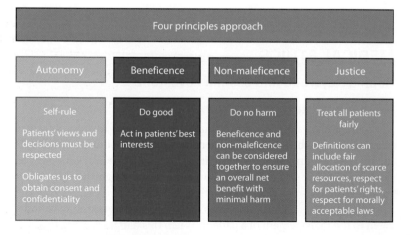

Figure 8.1 Four principles approach.

At medical school

Course content

As ethics teaching is a core component of all medical degrees, there will already be lectures, seminars and possibly small group workshops built into the curriculum. These sessions give students a chance to debate and start thinking critically about a wide range of topics. The easiest way to develop your interest in ethics is to make the most of the opportunities already laid out for you. So try to engage with these sessions, they are much more interesting and enjoyable this way.

Student-selected components and intercalation

There are times during the medical degree when students can specialise to a certain extent. Why not use this opportunity for ethics? Ethics is a subject that only gets more interesting the further you explore, so use these chances to get really stuck into a topic that interests you. Bristol and Birmingham offer BScs in medical ethics and King's College London has a BA in medical philosophy programme.

Electives

Most medical schools have the opportunity of an elective where you can spend a few weeks to a month specialising in an area of medicine you are interested in. You could use this time to either explore the academic world of medical ethics at a university institution or perhaps dive right in and see if you can shadow a hospital ethical board where daily decisions are made when ethical issues arise. If you are in the United Kingdom, the Institute of Medical Ethics (IME) awards bursaries for students who choose ethics as their elective specialty.

Extracurricular

Not only medical students and doctors are interested in medical ethics; it is a subject that fascinates the general public too. Cast your net beyond campus, and you will be sure to find talks or museum and gallery exhibits that explore issues relating to medical ethics. Get involved with the medical ethics society at your medical school. If there is not one already in place – set it up! This can be a fun, informal way to talk about ethics and share experiences with other students and a great excuse to invite interesting speakers who may well remember you later in your career.

Some ideas for events:

- Forums to discuss ethical cases from clinical placements
- Guest speakers
- Debates
- Revision events
- Conference trips (the IME has two annual conferences at which students are welcome, and they also host other ethics events you could attend)

Anecdote: Be patient in your society's early days

The first event of our newly formed medical ethics society was a speed dating-style debating event. We planned for weeks and had 30 people 'attending' on Facebook. Pizzas were ordered, the room was set up and we waited, but only two people came. Of course, we were very disappointed at first but in the end, this small group (six committee members and two guests) formed a good discussion, and we still had a great evening.

Future career impact and relevance

Medical ethics has the potential to open doors further on in a medical career. There is the obvious link to law for starters – an interest in medical ethics could lead on to a career in medical law later down the line. As discussed earlier in this book, some doctors undertake a law degree to become doubly qualified medicolegal lawyers. Medical ethics is also a speciality in its own right. Clinical and research ethicists, although few in number, are an essential part of the wider multidisciplinary organisation of healthcare.

Specialising purely in ethics is of course the extreme, but all doctors can find a way to incorporate an interest in ethics into their practice. Hospital ethics committees are a team of doctors, nurses, lawyers and other healthcare professionals. Subject to application and acceptance, a place on one of these committees could be a highlight of a career – with a chance to assist others in making the most difficult decisions in medicine. Ethics can be a highly academic discipline, but the most widespread ethics career for doctors is involvement in ethics education for medical students and junior doctors.

There is so much to learn in a medical degree that sometimes the importance of medical ethics is overlooked. Who has time to have a 30-minute debate when they have also to learn the mechanism of action of five different diabetic drugs and 12 cranial nerves? Yet medical ethics is everywhere in medicine. Starting to think more in depth about ethical decision-making at medical school will set a strong foundation for your future career as a doctor.

Engaging with medical ethics also allows you to explore a different side to medicine and develop different skills. During your medical career, you will be required to complete appraisals and portfolios. It is useful to understand the principles of medical ethics for these tasks. Embrace this opportunity to think creatively and explore different points of view – an invaluable skill for reflective practice.

Further afield

The key here is to keep aware of arising opportunities and be proactive! Medical schools are often contacted with information to circulate to students about conferences, prizes and committees to join. So skim through those e-mails, take a second glance at that poster and do not let a great opportunity pass you by.

Publications and prizes

There are many academic opportunities within medical ethics, similar to any other medical speciality. Look out for conferences to submit abstracts for posters and publications. Medical ethics institutions often hold essay competitions that are worth entering. Also, other groups such as the Royal Colleges or other national associations hold essay competitions. The themes, although under another speciality, may have an ethical twist you might find yourself in a good position to answer.

National committees

There will be some student societies run by governing bodies, for example, the IME. These may be student-only groups or student representative positions.

Hospital ethics committees

Most hospitals will have an ethics committee of some description – likely tied into the UK Clinical Ethics Network. This is usually a multidisciplinary team of doctors, lawyers, nurses and others. Often there

Top tips

1. *Speak up! Do not be shy –* The beauty of medical ethics is that there is no definite right and wrong answer so do not be afraid to share your opinions.
2. *Keep a reflective journal on placement –* This can help you remember interesting cases that come up and is a good habit for future reflective practice (i.e. appraisals).
3. *Current affairs –* Keep up to date with hot topics in the news and use them as an opportunity to think critically about your own ideas.
4. *Get talking! Everyone loves a good debate –* It may surprise you how many people have an opinion about medical issues, both medics and non-medics.

is a medical student representative. This is one of the rare opportunities when students can get involved in real-life ethics and have the opportunity to be involved in difficult decision-making for some of the most complicated cases in the hospital. Of course, places on these committees may be rare and competitive to get onto – so as with most aspects of medicine – being proactive and keen is the key.

Debating

There are networks in place for intermedical school debating. Think about putting a team together and entering.

Common pitfalls

1. *Be careful what you post online.*

   There is a growing online conversation about medical ethics, especially on Twitter. This is great to encourage wider discussion about ethics and current affairs but be wary of what you post. Remember that controversial statements could resurface in unfortunate situations in the future.

Further reading

Books:

BMA Ethics Department. *Everyday Medical Ethics and Law.* Wiley-Blackwell, Hoboken, NJ, 2013.

Hope, R. A., Savulescu, J., and Hendrick, J. *Medical Ethics and Law: The Core Curriculum,* 2nd Edition. Churchill Livingstone, London, 2008.

Papanikitas, A. *Crash Course: Medical Ethics and Sociology,* 2nd Edition. Mosby Ltd., Maryland Heights, MO, 2015.

Journals:

British Medical Journal and *Student British Medical Journal* – Good sources for discussion

Journal of Medical Ethics

Websites:

UK Clinical Ethics Network. http://www.ukcen.net. Accessed on October 17, 2017.

LEARNING TO TEACH

In-Ae Tribe with Jenny Higham

Background

To teach or not to teach – that is the question. There are many reasons to consider teaching while at medical school. It can help develop your understanding of a subject and lets you demonstrate your communication, time management and leadership skills. As a doctor, it forms part of your professional development and is ever present in your clinical job where you may find yourself teaching – or being taught by – colleagues, students and patients. Without doubt, enabling the learning of other students and sharing your specialist interests is a thoroughly rewarding and satisfying experience. However, learning how to become a *good* teacher takes time, practise and preparation with many resources now available. This section will describe how to get involved during medical school and how to make the most of the experiences.

Anecdote: Win–Win

I find teaching a great way to prepare for exams, by helping solidify and improve my understanding of a topic. Long hours of reading in a library can be fairly monotonous, but the didactic interaction in a teaching setting is much more fun. Create a study group and teach each other. Something must have worked as I passed my finals!

What makes a good teacher?

Irrespective of personal preference, good teachers possess a common set of traits. They will have an ability to clearly communicate, are well

VARK learning styles

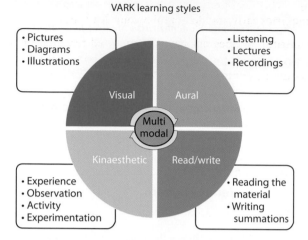

Figure 8.2   VARK model. (Courtesy of Velpic, Subiaco, Australia.)

organised and creative in adapting their material to suit and enthuse their students and will have sound knowledge of their teaching subject. Try to remember these when developing your own teaching style. Remember, there are many learning styles and your aim is to cater to the many during a session, in order to connect with the whole audience. Try to incorporate the visual, auditory, reading and kinaesthetic (VARK) model [1] by using images, words, video and kinetic elements such as role play or doing tasks (see Figure 8.2). This enables you to identify your own areas of weakness that may require more effort in order to accommodate for all learner preferences, e.g. providing more images/diagrams rather than text.

Getting involved at medical school

Medical school is an ideal environment to become involved in teaching: your skills are immediately transferrable to earlier years; your training is largely standardised; and there are many students eager to learn. Your first step should be to look at what is already set up to achieve this. Some universities have their own peer-teaching sessions where senior students can facilitate small group teaching on prepared curricular material. Such programmes will probably offer training and feedback, which is very helpful for new teachers starting out. You may also have the chance to earn some money at the same time (some institutions pay students to be peer tutors). But take note, structured peer-led teaching programmes often require an application process – make enquiries early and do not miss your deadlines.

If your institution does not have a structured teaching programme, or if you are looking for something more ad hoc – consider how you could set up a teaching scheme. Often universities have a variety of specialty specific societies from radiology to surgery to paediatrics. If you have a particular interest, why not join their committee to influence teaching events or offer to lecture their members on a topic? All medical schools have a form of student medical education committee (often requiring representatives from each year group) – this is a great opportunity to see how a medical school curriculum is put together.

Alternatively, you could set up your own revision sessions independent from a society or group, although this needs proper planning:

1. Select which year group to teach and a suitable date in their calendar.
2. Decide on the length of your programme: weekly lecture series vs. intense course.
3. Decide how you want to deliver the revision material: lectures, small group teaching, mock role play?
4. Finally, select and find people qualified to help you teach.
5. Follow up with participants and compile feedback.

However, if public speaking is not your thing (see Chapter 4), there are other ways you can teach, including through recorded lectures or podcasts and revision notes or questions. There are many websites and groups that offer opportunities for you to contribute notes or questions as a writer; see 'Further reading' section for more details.

How to teach

It is not easy to know how best to teach; this is a skill that takes years to develop. There are a range of approaches you can use to help guide you; a commonly used example is the Danielson Framework [2]. Applying this to teaching at medical school essentially, it boils down to three main components:

1. Planning and preparation stage
2. 'On the job' stage
3. Reflection and professional development

Planning and preparation

If you are teaching in a session which has tutor notes already written (by academic staff or students), make sure that you have read through these. Prepare by highlighting key words that will prompt your memory of important points students need to learn. Plan by picturing how the session will flow, with logical transitions from one topic to the next. This includes what materials/images you might want to show students to help explain or illustrate difficult concepts.

If you are writing your own material, make sure that you always work from the mantra of 'know your target audience'. This will guide you in deciding what material to cover, in what detail and how best to deliver it. There is no point turning up to first-year medical students – mere tadpoles in the great lake of medicine – and asking them to perform a full examination of a real-life clinically unwell patient. This prior consideration is vital in gauging the length of time to teach and keeping what you cover applicable to your students and their learning objectives. As a student, you are bombarded by information which can make knowing what to learn difficult. As a teacher, you are there to help filter – providing an overview and explanation of the key learning elements of a topic, such that students can deepen their knowledge on their own.

When preparing your material, treat it as though it is a story with a beginning, middle and end: Start with the contents or learning objectives so students know what to expect. Then, contextualise the topic for them. Why is this session important to them? How will this build on their prior knowledge? For example, if you are teaching about pancreatitis, it is worth actually mentioning what the pancreas does to ensure they understand the wider pathology and principles of management (you would be surprised how this can be overlooked). Check with students what they already know about your subject. This can guide you in knowing how detailed you can be with explanations and might relax the mood and calm student nerves to engage.

By the middle of the session, you will want to be in full flow. This is where you will

Top tip: Catering to the many

Have additional questions you can ask for those students who seem to whittle quickly through the provided material. Alternatively, another tactic is recapping what you have covered. Repetition and recall is helpful for students to retain the information they have learnt.

deliver the bulk of the teaching material. Make sure your transitions through the material are logical and chunk information to aid your students in committing it to memory. If using a slideshow, try not to simply read from the slide – have concise points that act as prompts and use pictures or diagrams to show what you are explaining. As you come towards conclusion, prepare to summarise what you have discussed and give your students two or three key learning points or 'take-home messages', and be ready to signpost them to where they can access good resources for independent learning. The final part of preparation is ensuring that you have all the materials you need: think about what equipment you require, the size and setup of the room that you will have and how you will access it on the day. Do not be caught out – get to your teaching session early, there is nothing worse than a tardy *and* sweaty teacher!

'On the job'

Creating the right learning environment is central to ensuring the session runs smoothly. Hence, start by introducing yourself; explain who you are and how you want the session to run. Ask yourself what is the culture of the teaching session – informal or formal? You may wish to let the group introduce themselves too if it is not too big. When delivering the content, adjust it based on whether it is the first time students have heard the material or whether it is a revision. If it is the former, you may wish to give more information than you ask of your students; however, if it is a revision – try challenging them through questions and recall.

Engage the *whole* audience, being considerate to the diversity within the group. If you are in a small group, try to ensure that everyone answers a question. Going round a group makes it fairer, as there will always be someone who can't stop talking. However, if someone is struggling, do not let them stew – open it up to the floor for help or consider having students discuss answers with the person next to them prior to sharing as a group, which may encourage the shyer individuals to engage. Assessment can be another approach of engaging. Having a quiz with multiple choice questions can be a good way to get students thinking and push them to recall their knowledge. If there is time, short tasks such as splitting a group into pairs to practise a skill can be another way to create a didactic learning session. Time management is key; do not lose focus. Research suggests that a person's attention span is no longer than 20 minutes, so try chunking material with

Top tip: Adapting to your audience

If you think your audience already know a great deal about your subject material, you can try to change the delivery of your teaching. For example, by asking them questions of the material that might be on the next slide: e.g. what investigations would you carry out next? Why? At every stage, you should aim to be adaptive to your students' knowledge and abilities.

breaks or keeping sessions short [3]. Going too fast or too slow may leave topics covered inadequately, so pace yourself and wear a watch. Talking in front of a crowd can be difficult but breaking your material up into sections can give you breathing points too. Keep a time schedule with a bit of slack so you can keep track during the session. Do not be afraid of the '5-minute break' – sometimes a quick sip of water and a few minutes of downtime can give you and the students some respite. While they consolidate the information you have given them, you have the chance to check that all is in order as you head towards ending the session.

Personal and professional development

As mentioned earlier, teaching is core to your future career development. However, if you want this to be recognised by others, you need to provide evidence of what you have done. This can come in a range of forms: certificates from the society or university who organised the session, your own teaching materials, participant feedback sheets and so on. There is also an expectation in postgraduate education that teachers are somewhat 'qualified' to teach, with many courses designed to 'train the trainer', but these are costly and for consideration if you choose to pursue a career in clinical education. Common qualifications in the United Kingdom include the Post Graduate Certificate in Education and its variations such as clinical and medical education and master's of medical education courses.

Further, self-reflection will improve your sessions and help you become a better teacher, so get in the habit of keeping a logbook of what you have done. Include dates, the type and number of participants and keep a handout of your slides or other material produced. Ensure you have feedback forms and reflect on these and the session as a whole. A short reflective paragraph will help you consolidate your thoughts; include details such as what you taught, what went well, what could have gone better and what you will do differently next time. Doing this regularly will not only improve your teaching skills but can serve as strong evidence of your professionalism to be included in your portfolio for future jobs. Another helpful form of feedback can be gained from peers or personal tutors observing your sessions.

Case study: From educator to principal
Jenny Higham

What advice would I give to my colleagues who are closer to graduation? Keep nimble and keep your options open! I never saw myself as an academic on graduation – I thought I was straightforward NHS teaching hospital material, but life evolved down a very different route. Opportunities arouse, and I had a tendency always to say yes and this lead to a bigger and bigger thing – just before my consultant level appointment, the new medical school of Imperial was being created out of the former Charing Cross and Westminster – and St Mary's schools. I had always enjoyed education and so was happy to wade into negotiating the Obstetrics and Gynaecology curriculum between the two sides (who were both convinced that theirs was best!). From that small start, my career in education grew and grew – to eventually being the medical school head at Imperial College London and opening a new medical school in Singapore. I now have a brilliant new challenge, in charge of a university. I have travelled, learnt a great deal, still managed to keep practicing clinically and, most importantly, never been bored!

Making money

As a medical student, it can be difficult to earn money due to the constraints of course contact time or self-study. Teaching is one of the few things you can do while at medical school and be paid for it. This will be most straightforward if your medical school pays students to teach. If not, you could contact an agency or go direct via self-advertisement, depending on your preference and availability. If you still recall your high school science, you may wish to tutor high school/senior school students sitting their exams. Alternatively, national courses run by student or professional organisations may recruit teachers and demonstrators, and this too could serve as a chance to earn some money. A long time ago, some medical students published their revision notes – the result of this is the *Oxford Clinical Handbook*. While there are still opportunities to publish educational books – this does not generally pay well as most medical books: the rewards are more intellectual!

Conclusion

Medical school provides ample opportunities to get involved in teaching and develop lifelong transferrable skills that you can build on and log for professional development. Teaching well requires time and preparation, but this can be rewarding both personally and financially. Do not forget 'know your target audience' and you will not go far wrong.

Common pitfalls

1. *'You have done too much, much too long'.*

    Trying to cover too much material in a short time frame is a great temptation; however, less is definitely more. Practise your presentations and try to create a timeline for when to finish which sections in order to keep you on track.

2. *'I had to wake one of my students up'.*

    Firm engagement is key. If you have an audience not willing to communicate, try dividing the room and picking someone from each part to answer. Adding in personal experience and anecdotes can make the material more appealing.

3. *'Computer says no'.*

    Have plans B and C for digital failure. Store slides in two electronic locations, e.g. a USB stick and online/cloud storage. Be careful if you think your location might have safeguards to non-encrypted devices and always print your slides as a hard copy. If technology fails (like it is wanton to do), think on your feet and use your hard copy backup as prompts.

References

1. VARK Learn Limited. *Introduction to VARK*. 2016. http://vark-learn.com /introduction-to-vark/the-vark-modalities/. Accessed on June 14, 2017.

2. Danielson Group. *The Framework*. 2013. https://www.danielsongroup .org/framework/. Accessed on June 14, 2017.

3. Dukette, D., and Cornish, D. *The Essential 20: Twenty Components of an Excellent Health Care Team*, pp. 72–3. Rose Dog Books, Pittsburgh, PA, 2009.

Further reading

For further instruction on teaching theory and practise:

Cantillon, P. and Wood, D. *ABC of Learning and Teaching in Medicine*, 2nd Edition. Wiley, Hoboken, NJ, 2010.

McKimm, J., Forrest, K. and Thistlewaite, J. *Wiley Medical Education at a Glance*, 1st Edition. Wiley, Hoboken, NJ, 2017.

For medical revision notes where you can contribute as author:

Almostadoctor. http://almostadoctor.co.uk/.

Fastbleep. http://www.fastbleep.com/revision-notes/get-involved.

To become a podstar check out:

Podlearn. http://www.podlearn.org/.

Podmedics. https://www.podmedics.com/.

For further details on postgraduate education in medicine:

Higher Education Academy. https://www.heacademy.ac.uk.

Search university courses and programmes hosted by the Royal Colleges.

CHAPTER 9

Trading places
Medicine abroad

CONTENTS

STUDYING MEDICINE ABROAD

Wong Yisheng

Background

In this day and age of globalisation, the dream of studying medicine can be realised like never before. Studying medicine abroad is becoming increasingly common as medical schools seek to cater to a global medical cohort, often with training split across different countries. This chapter aims to allay any uncertainties and provide you with a practical step-by-step guide on how to prepare and succeed in studying part or all of medicine in a different country.

Why study medicine abroad?

There are a variety of reasons why one would want to study medicine abroad. University years may be one of the most formative periods during our lifetime, shaping our personal and professional development. Spending these years overseas helps to broaden your horizon – you get to make friends from different countries, explore new places and cultures and, most importantly, gain a whole new life experience. With studying medicine a highly competitive endeavour, you may be forced to consider this route if your national options are limited.

Before deciding

Despite all the attractive benefits of studying medicine abroad, there are a range of factors to consider before making your decision.

Finance

Medicine is one of the most expensive courses in any university. For international students, the fees can be vastly increased compared to domestic students, making the study of medicine overseas very expensive. For example, UK fees per annum for international students are in the order of fivefold higher than those for UK students. There is a need to take into account the length of the course (and the increased fees during the clinical years), as well as the costs of living.

Logistics

For many students, this may be the first considerable period away from home. Studying abroad will throw you out of your comfort zone, quickly forcing you to become independent; and while medicine can be a whole lot of fun, it is also sometimes stressful. On top of that, you need to be prepared to deal with searching for your own accommodation, grocery shopping for your daily needs, the laundry etc. You will also be leaving your family and friends that you are so used to being with back home. Vacation breaks may only go so far to reliving home sickness.

Deciding where to go

There are over 2000 medical schools in 180 countries. So one of your first questions will be where should I go? Do some research and start planning ahead. Envision yourself 5–10 years down the road. Would you prefer to work in your home country or are you an adventurous soul set on settling down abroad? This is important because each country has a list of acceptable primary medical qualifications. Therefore, take some time to enquire with the medical council of your country (for example, General Medical Council in the United Kingdom) regarding the list of medical degrees that meet their set acceptability criteria. In general, the more reputable the medical school, the more internationally recognised the medical degree conferred will be.

Course requirements and structure

Another important consideration is to fully understand the entry requirements for the medical schools that you are applying to. Medical schools require a certain set of grades, interviews, entry examinations, referee letters etc. Download a university prospectus to learn more. If you cannot find it, do not be shy – send an e-mail to the admissions tutor with your enquiry. Make sure you have fulfilled or will be able to fulfil the requirements by the application closing date.

Before applying to medical schools, there is a need to understand the variety of programmes offered. There is a difference between undergraduate and graduate programmes. In the United States, entry into medical school requires an undergraduate degree, whereas in the United Kingdom or Australia, there is a mix of both undergraduate and graduate courses for medicine. The lengths of programmes differ as well, ranging from a 4-year graduate course to a 6-year programme with an optional (or for some institutions, compulsory) intercalated degree. For those budding clinician-scientists, there are even medical schools offering MBBS/PhD or MD/PhD routes which can take up to 9 years.

Language

Language is an important factor in deciding where to go. Although most medical schools use English as a medium of teaching, you need to understand that once you get into the clinical years, you will need to interact with patients. If you are not intending to learn a whole new language, I would not recommend a country in which you do not speak its native language at all. However, if you are a talented multilinguist, this should not be an issue. Further, some medical schools may require you to take a language proficiency test if English is not your native language (e.g. International English Language Testing System for UK medical schools).

Applying
Entrance examinations

Depending on which medical schools you apply for, there may be prerequisite entrance examinations that you have to pass before application. Examples would be the BMAT or the UK Clinical Aptitude Test required for some medical schools in the United Kingdom. Some Australian medical schools will require the Undergraduate Medicine and Health Sciences Admission Test. It is important to understand the components of these entrance examinations, and there are various resources online to help prepare for them. These examinations often test higher-order thinking abilities such as logical reasoning, decision-making and sometimes quantitative reasoning.

Interviews

Medical school interviews are often the most nerve-wrecking and feared part of the application process. But it is important to understand that having secured an interview is already half the battle won. Most medical schools will require face-to-face interviews with prospective students, but some may give potential international students the option of an interview via a different medium, e.g. Skype.

Preparation for the medical school interview is important. Firstly, know the format of the interview. Some medical schools still use the traditional interview method of questions and answers in front of an interview panel; others use the format of multiple mini interviews, where applicants spend an allocated amount of time in role play or open questioning at various stations. The scenarios often evaluate soft skills such as empathy, ethical reasoning, communications skills etc. They also test for your problem-solving abilities. Most stations will involve an actor whom you are expected to interact with and an interviewer who will be observing you working through the station. Although this form of interview seems daunting, most candidates report finding it enjoyable (in retrospect!).

Remember that what interviewers are looking out for is whether you would be someone whom a patient would feel comfortable and safe with. Box 9.1 contains some top tips (not exhaustive) for a successful interview.

Box 9.1   Interview tips

- Dress presentably.
- Be punctual.
- Keep calm.
- Be polite, shake hands and maintain eye contact.
- Be enthusiastic and positive.
- Clear and concise communication.
- Be prepared but do not appear overrehearsed.
- Expect the unexpected and be flexible.

Planning your escape

Congratulations in getting a place in a medical school abroad! Planning for your big transition requires time. It is never too early to plan ahead. It would be helpful to create a checklist to ease your transition before departure.

Finances

Studying medicine abroad requires financial commitment. Medical school fees for international students vary according to different medical schools and can be significantly higher than what local students pay. They are also often increased during the clinical years compared to pre-clinical years. It is important to note that financial aid or scholarships for international medical students are rare. You also need to factor in costs of living including accommodation, daily living expenses for food, transportation, entertainment etc. Open a bank account early – certain banks allow you to open an account even when you are still in your home country.

Travel

Book your flight for arrival at least a week before your course begins if time permits. This will give you time to settle in, adapt to the new environment (or weather), orientate yourself and make some friends before the semester starts.

Find a buddy

Some countries have networks which bring together medical students who will be going abroad, some even providing orientation activities locally before departure. These networks are valuable resources as seniors may provide you with important tips pertaining to 'surviving the new habitat', especially as an international student. It helps to have a strong social network overseas as you will never know when you may need help or feel homesick. These people may become your lifelong friends.

Administrative issues

There are many other miscellaneous administrative tasks that you may need to do pre-departure. This includes ensuring your insurance covers your stint overseas, ensuring that your passport is valid and ensuring that you have applied for a visa (if necessary).

Learn the culture

Borrow or purchase a reliable travel guide that introduces you to the country/region that you are going to. Make an effort to learn about the culture. This will also be beneficial in your communication and interaction with patients during your course.

Making the transition and succeeding

Adapting to a whole new country and culture can be daunting even for the most extroverted of people. There are a few tips which can make this transition a whole lot easier.

- Stay at the university dormitories/campus housing in the first year. This is a chance to get to mingle with your peers, no matter whether they are locals or international students. There are often activities and events organised within the dormitories which are a perfect opportunities to establish new relationships. Forming a social network early on will allow a more smooth-sailing transition.

- Join the international students' society (it may be named differently) in your university as getting advice from veterans (senior international students) who had been in your position before can be very reassuring.

- Form a study group early on. As a first-year medical student adapting to a whole new environment, there is no shame in asking questions – so ask whenever you are in doubt. Some universities provide international students with mentors within the faculty. Meet up with your mentor often to track your progress. However, do not forget to have fun.

- Most universities have a variety of interest groups, so feel free to join a few and make new friends. Attend social events, explore the city during the weekends and make sure you make the most of your time abroad.

Returning back home or staying?

The decision of returning back home or staying after graduation is a very personal one. If you are unsure, it would be helpful to apply for clinical electives in your home country during the holidays to get a taste of how it is working back home. You will then be able to compare the work culture and make a more informed decision. A more thorough analysis of practising overseas is included in the next chapter.

Conclusion

Moving abroad to study medicine may be a daunting idea to some people. However, it could be one of the best decisions, as long as you know what to expect and how to prepare for it. Good luck!

Common pitfalls and how to overcome them

1. Not considering studying medicine abroad because it is 'out of your comfort zone': This is doing yourself a huge disfavour.
2. It is perfectly normal to feel homesick abroad, but do pick yourself up and make the most out of your overseas experience.
3. Not adapting to the culture of the country you are in: Keep an open mind and seek out support from seniors or other international students.
4. Managing of finances for students is tough, but being abroad may make it even more difficult. Financial planning for daily expenses is important.

Further reading

Acceptable overseas medical qualifications by the General Medical Council. http://www.gmc-uk.org/doctors/registration_applications/acceptable_primary _medical qualification.asp.

Applying to medical schools in UK. http://www.medschools.ac.uk/Students /howtoapply/international/Pages/default.aspx.

Stone-Brown, K., and Spreadbury, M. Should you study medicine abroad? *Student BMJ*. http://student.bmj.com/student/view-article.html?id=sbmj .g1694.

Studying in Australia's medical schools. https://ama.com.au/careers /becoming-a-doctor.

PRACTISING MEDICINE ABROAD

Randa ElMallah

Background

There are many factors that go into deciding where to go to practice after medical school. Often personal circumstances, such as family, spouses, and such else, influence the decision. Alternatively, certain academic or work aspirations, such as lifestyle, academia or method of training drive international relocation. Regardless of your reason, having a stepwise and organised approach can make the crucial difference between securing a spot in a competitive residency/training programme or joining the long list of unsuccessful applicants. The purpose of this section is to outline key steps to successfully securing a position to practice medicine abroad. It draws on the author's experience of securing a residency position in the United States. However, the following steps can be broadly applied to medical students wishing to practice medicine anywhere abroad.

Planning your escape: A 3-year strategy

Such a significant transition requires considerable planning, often years ahead. For transition to the United States, obtaining a residency position as an *international graduate* is particularly difficult and requires a considerably higher degree of effort than most American applicants. Unlike in the United Kingdom, where most doctors can decide on their specialty throughout foundation training, those applying abroad must choose their specialty far in advance. Firstly, you must decide the subspecialty you wish to choose. After this, research the requirements for admission either through programme materials online or via direct contact with physicians, as each has different entry requirements. Having an idea of these requirements may aid in setting realistic goals for the milestones ahead including building your network, licensing examinations and interviews.

Taking a UK-to-US transition as an example, the training process to become a licensed doctor in the United States is called residency. As mentioned earlier, medical students enter straight into their specialty of choosing, i.e. orthopaedic surgery, without doing the foundation training that is required in the United Kingdom. Residency begins in July of each year, but the application process starts in September the year before. Bear this in mind as you prepare your application; I have seen many applicants defer their application because of not realising how early the process begins.

Examinations

A transition exam is often required, and it goes without saying that to be a competitive applicant, performing well on these exams is vital. For the United States, all medical students (American and international) need to sit the US Medical Licensing Examination (USMLE). This consists of three parts or steps. The first step consists of basic science topics, which are often covered in the early years of medical school and in the first 2 years of the 5-year UK and European medical school systems. The USMLE step 1 exam is often considered to be the most difficult one, and the score obtained in this exam is often the most important defining factor in the selection process. This is especially true when applying to surgical specialties. If you are utilising the 3-year escape strategy mentioned earlier, then a significant proportion of your early planning is dedicated to this step of the exam. However, even if you are planning on practicing in less than 3 years, I would highly recommend focussing considerable effort on doing well in this exam, which depending on personal study techniques, can take up to 3 months of preparation.

The second USMLE consists of two portions, a written clinical and a practical exam (CS). These are much more clinically orientated and are often considered to be a little less challenging. As an international applicant, a high score on the written exam is essential, and again, considerable effort and time to study may be necessary. The practical exam consists of clinical stations, with real-life or acting patients. You take the role of a physician and are required to take a history, perform the relevant examinations, communicate a differential diagnosis and write a clinical note encompassing the investigations and the further management necessary. However, this practical exam is only a pass/fail and is not score dependent.

A trap that many people fall into with the step 2 clinical skills examination (CS) is not booking it early enough. To be a competitive applicant, it is recommended to have all your scores ready by the application date (usually mid-September). Because most medical students applying are aiming to do this, all the available slots are often taken as early as June. It is important to consider this and either book early or take the exam as early as March or April of the application year, particularly as testing centres are only available in select cities.

Traditionally, step 3 is taken during the first year of residency. However, there is much debate about whether or not an international applicant should take this prior to applying. I am often on the fence about this and think that it depends on three factors: (1) the programme you are applying to, (2) your visa status and (3) if you have enough preparation time to do well on it.

1. If the programme you are interested in requires that international graduates complete this exam prior to matching, then the decision is easy and you should factor this exam into your application timeline.

2. If you are an American citizen or a green card holder, then your visa status does not factor into whether or not you should take this. However, if you are deciding between a J-1 or H-1 visa, doing the exam may influence your ability to get one. I would recommend looking into this early in your application process.

3. If you do not have visa restrictions or the programmes do not specify whether or not they would like you to do the step 3, then the decision is often less clear. Many advocate that doing it prior to starting residency will enhance your application as an international graduate. However, I feel that this exam can both hurt and help you. If you feel that you can dedicate enough time to do well on this prior to application, then you may consider taking it. If you cannot dedicate the necessary time to the examination to obtain an above average score, I would recommend against doing it. A poor score on step 3 is more likely to negatively impact your application than not taking it at all. Personally, I did not feel like I could dedicate the time prior to applying to do well on it, so I postponed it until after I matched into a programme.

Anecdote: Scoring high

Given the disadvantage international graduates are at, scoring highly in these examinations can be a defining factor in their application. This is becoming more obvious as many residency programmes are now providing cut-off scores for applications to certain competitive specialties. For example, the step 1 cut-off for applications to orthopaedic residency can be as high as 245–250 for programme directors to even consider your application.

Letters of recommendation

Obtaining letters of recommendations (LORs) can occur prior to or after sitting entrance exams. Getting these should be on your mind early in the application process. For the United States, many programmes are often more interested in receiving at least one to two LORs from American physicians. However, doing this as an international applicant is difficult as clinical rotations are often done in an applicant's home country. Thus, if possible, it is recommended you undertake some of your clinical rotations abroad in the country you wish to practice in. This will aid you to both secure an LOR from a physician native to that country – and begin to build connections in the country where you would like to practice.

To get an LOR in the United States, you will often have to spend time rotating at a programme, usually for a month. You can do this as a clerkship/subinternship (sub-i), where you are allowed to scrub into surgeries and participate in clinical care or as an observer, where you are not allowed to have patient contact. The first is obviously better, particularly when you are trying to get an LOR from someone who is assessing your medical skills. However, obtaining a sub-i is significantly more difficult, and you can only do this if you are still a medical student (hence, why you need to plan way in advance of graduation!). Doing a rotation abroad as a medical student strengthens your LOR and therefore your application considerably more than if you are already a graduate and can only observe. However, doing an observership can still be helpful. Regardless of whether you are aiming to get a sub-i or an observership, you often have to apply for this a few months in advance. I would highly recommend doing your rotation at a hospital that has a residency programme, that has accepted international graduates before and that you would consider practicing/matching at. You should aim to have all your reference letters, or LORs, compiled by the application opening date.

Ticking boxes

As mentioned earlier, after appropriately researching your specialty of choice, setting realistic goals is mandatory. This involves deciding whether you are able or willing to tick all the necessary boxes. Aside from successfully completing any entrance examinations, you must start assembling the other components of your application.

An up-to-date CV is your first step. Minor details, such as formatting it correctly, ensuring consistent font etc., are important – I have sat on several committees where CVs have automatically been dismissed based on these factors. This may seem unfair, but when it comes to dealing with hundreds of overqualified applicants, board members and interviewers look for anything to help differentiate them – and an unpolished CV is one of them. If in any doubt about the content or format, ask several of your peers to critique it. As you build on your experiences and take the required examinations, you should update your CV periodically until your application day. Additional achievements are also highly regarded such as research experience, publications, clinical awards and so on. Factoring these into your application strategy plan will strengthen your submission.

Depending on where you are applying, a personal statement or a description of yourself and your interest in the specialty you are pursuing may be required. As this is a personal reflection of yourself, this can be approached in a multitude of ways. However, it is imperative that you get at least one or two trusted peers to edit and critique this. Finally, when your application has been compiled, make sure this is reviewed by yourself and ideally a supervisor or mentor familiar with the application system you are pursuing.

If at first you do not succeed

Failure is difficult, regardless of the situation. But this need not be a huge problem, particularly if you know what steps are necessary to succeed the next time. Unfortunately, in such a gruelling application process, you have to be 100% committed. So ask yourself: Do you still want to make the transition abroad? And if so, are you still settled on a specific specialty?

If the answer to these questions is yes, then you have two options:

1. Doing a preliminary or transitional year
2. Doing research

Preliminary or transitional year

Many programmes have 1-year positions, either a preliminary year in general surgery or a transitional year in internal medicine. These are similar to the non-training clinical fellow posts becoming more common in the United Kingdom. Although these are paid positions, you are not in a categorical residency programme, which is a straight track to an attending or consultant position, and you have to reapply for a position the following year.

The advantage of these positions are as follows:

1. You are getting paid.
2. You are a practicing physician.

3. You may have the opportunity to either rotate in the specialty you are interested in or build connections with doctors in the department you want to match in.

However, not all programmes will offer these benefits. Focus on those which have a residency programme and offer the chance to spend a month or two in the desired specialty. The major disadvantage of this year is that you may not have added a great deal to your application apart from a couple of months of clinical experience. When making your decision ask yourself, colleagues and prospective employers the questions in Box 9.2.

Box 9.2 Deciding on a transitional year

1. What are the opportunities for me to rotate in (insert desired specialty) while I am working this year?
2. How many people that have taken this position have matched into (insert desired specialty)?
3. What opportunities do you provide for people who do not match following this year/what have people done who have not matched following this year?

I appreciate that these questions may seem direct and borderline blunt, but it is better for you to find these out early, and programmes often respect and appreciate an applicant who is direct with and confident about what he or she wants.

Research fellowships

In choosing to undertake a research fellowship, you are looking for an opportunity to improve your CV for the next application cycle. Consider the application timeline of the country you are applying to. For example, in the United States, you find out whether you have been accepted onto a programme in March. Should you elect to begin a research fellowship in July, you will only have 3 months before the application cycle for next year begins (in September). For this reason, fellowships are often 2-year commitments to allow you enough time to publish before you apply the following cycle – see Box 9.3 for the pros and cons.

Box 9.3   Pros and cons of a research fellowship

✓ You have an opportunity to publish and build your CV in a way most applicants do not.

✓ You can build connections with the department and specialty you are interested in.

✗ You are not guaranteed a publication.

✗ The research fellowship may not have any connections to a residency programme.

As the competitiveness of matching into residency continuously increases, the number of research fellowships available in different specialties has exponentially grown. Many of these cater to unsuccessful applicants looking to match in the future. However, the quality of these programmes can vary. Again, ask the questions in Box 9.4.

Box 9.4   Deciding on a research fellowship

---

1. What are my chances of matching at (your desired specialty) programme?
2. How many applicants have you successfully matched at a programme at your institution or at others?
3. What are my chances of actually publishing a paper prior to the next application cycle?
4. How many papers do research fellows average during this 2-year commitment?

Anecdote: Perseverance and strategy

I did not match when I first applied for my desired specialty in the United States. I was devastated, but I knew that this was what I wanted to pursue. I chose to undertake a research fellowship, as I think there are more opportunities available for you to maximise and strengthen your application. After completing my 2-year fellowship, I matched into orthopaedic surgery; I do not think I would have if it were not for my achievements and the connections that I made during those 2 years. Note that I was very direct in what I was looking for when choosing my research position and thus selected the one with the highest publication yield and successful match rate.

Making the transition and returning

You have successfully matched or obtained a position in the specialty and country of your choice! Now that the biggest hurdle is finally over, see Boxes 5.3 and 5.4 earlier in this book for the key issues to address when moving abroad. Making the move abroad can be permanent or temporary. It is difficult giving generic advice on this topic, as the ease of returning back home depends on the individual situation and the country. Returning back home to the United Kingdom after training in the United States or vice versa is difficult, as the training programmes are not equivalent, and often, applicants have to start over. In rare circumstances, doctors may undertake one or more years of focussed training, or clinical fellowships, to achieve a permanent consultant/attending position.

Conclusion

Making the decision to practice abroad can be a daunting one, and the journey can be long and harrowing. However, the benefits of experiencing new places, meeting new people and fulfilling your professional dream often make this worth it. Regardless of your reason for making the move, it is important to remember that there is a network of other internationals who have done the same and who are willing to provide you with the support and advice you need.

Further reading

Chetwood, J. Foundation training overseas: How to apply and the pitfalls to avoid. *BMJ Careers*. 2015. http://careers.bmj.com/careers/advice/Foundation _training_overseas%3A_how_to_apply_and_the_pitfalls_to_avoid.

Meraj, A. Pursuing training in the United States. *BMJ Careers*. 2010. http:// careers.bmj.com/careers/advice/Pursuing_training_in_the_United_States.

Seymour, C. Working in another country. *BMJ Careers*. 2009. http://careers .bmj.com/careers/advice/Working_in_another_country.

Vest, A. R. Working in the US. *Student BMJ*. http://student.bmj.com/student /view-article.html?id=sbmj.b1064.

CHAPTER 10

Career perspectives

CONTENTS

SCIENCE

Babak Javid

The physician-scientist career is an accident of history – forged by late nineteenth- and early twentieth-century pioneers who bridged both disciplines. It can be the best of both worlds, but demands focus and dedication in the face of increasing administrative and financial obstacles to ensure career success. The life of physician-scientists involves a tricky balancing act. The vast majority of colleagues who dedicate their lives to clinical service think you 'play at being a doctor', while pure scientists resent the often higher salaries that physician-scientists make, especially in the training phase of the career. To top it all, given that the actual demands of both professions are so different, the time required for training in both is double that of someone specialising in just one, so one can be in one's forties before settling down.

So why should any young physician in training consider such a career? In my own case, it was a fascination with *not knowing*. Much of medical school involves memorising thousands of facts. We learn the steps of the Krebs cycle or oxidative phosphorylation, not realising that until they were discovered, there was nothing obvious about them, and indeed, in many cases, we still only have partial models explaining the natural world and disease processes. I became interested in the *gaps* more than the *facts*. Having superb mentors throughout my training career, as a medical student and as a young clinician helped me realise that I can forge a career in the business of *what we do not know*. The decision to go back to university to undertake a PhD halfway through my clinical training was very difficult, but one which I have never regretted. Life at the bench is very different to life at the bedside. The latter can not only be physically and mentally exhausting, but also involves instant gratification – your patient either gets better or worse, usually in a matter of days. Once you go off shift, someone else will carry the burden, at least to a large extent. The lab is the complete opposite. No one else will do your experiment, or thinking, if you do not. It just will not get done, ever. Even after having a *brilliant idea*, it can take months or years to develop the experimental assay that shows that it was not so brilliant after all or, sometimes, that there is an even more brilliant question waiting to be asked. Failure is the norm rather than the exception. I am a *professor*, but I only work on and get excited about those things I do not understand.

So, if *being ignorant* gets you excited, what can you do about it? The first piece of advice I would offer would be to dip your toe in the water whenever you get the chance. Yes, you do have to memorise the steps of the Krebs cycle, but that does not mean that you cannot be curious about the mystical *scientific process*. After all, almost all your lecturers and teachers will be engaging in science as well as or indeed instead of medicine. Secondly, summer vacations are a great time to engage in some supervised independent research. More and more of these opportunities are available today. It involves being organised: it is no good writing to a potential lab host 1 month before the summer begins, and it will involve forgoing the beach in Thailand with your best mates for a wooden bench, not so cool lab coat and over familiarity with a pipette. Most medical schools offer a variety of intercalated degrees. However, many of these options offer no or very limited opportunities for real fundamental research. Over the years, I have had countless medical students come to me and tell me that they want to do a library project for their intercalated year. There is nothing wrong with that per se, but I would counter that this is your one chance to do something different. I certainly had no inkling that I would end up on an academic track when I decided to study the *theory of mind* of 3-year-olds in Cambridge kindergartens, but it seemed like fun, so I went for it. Importantly, the fact that my early experience in research was in no way related to what I do now (genetics of *Mycobacterium tuberculosis* – the bacterium that causes tuberculosis) was no bar in terms of paving the way for a future academic career.

It might be argued that if one wants to be a scientist, why not just do that instead of also adding the decade and a half of medical training. I think that is a fair comment. Some of my colleagues argue that physician-scientists have a unique *clinical perspective* regarding which fundamental scientific questions are more likely to be important for human health and disease. While that may be true in a few individual cases, I do not think that it is generally true. Most of my scientist colleagues are exactly that – superb scientists. They do not need me to tell them which scientific questions are important to address. So does the world absolutely need physician-scientists? Truthfully, probably not. But that does not mean that the world does not benefit from having them around. And I can attest that being one is certainly a wonderful privilege and a huge amount of fun.

PUBLIC ENGAGEMENT

Frank Chinegwundoh

I have been fortunate to enjoy a wide-ranging career encompassing medicine (specifically urology), teaching, examining, voluntary sector, media work, international collaborations and much more. I was born in London in the 1960s to Nigerian parents who were first-generation immigrants – their mantra was education. Having attended a grammar school in London, I gained entry into St George's Hospital Medical School in London. That was a social eye-opener, mixing with students very much not from an inner-city experience. Once qualified as a doctor, I embarked on a surgical career and, after gaining a master of surgery degree by thesis, was accepted onto a specialist urology training programme. As a consultant, there is the opportunity to develop a specialty interest. I chose urological oncology and, in particular, prostate cancer.

Having observed many African–Caribbean men in my practice with prostate cancer, I had one research question in mind – was prostate cancer commoner in African men? Data from the United States suggested so. I was able to conduct a study in East London that published the first UK data demonstrating a two- to threefold higher incidence of prostate cancer in African men compared with Caucasian men. This led to media interest. Once you have a *name*, other opportunities arise. I was asked to become a trustee of a new charity in 1996, called Cancer Black Care (CBC). This was set up in Hackney, London, to provide support to African and ethnic minority cancer sufferers. I became chairman in 1998 and continue in that role. Through my work with CBC as well as my publications, I was invited to join a range of regional and national groups and bodies on prostate cancer.

As one's profile develops, media opportunities arise. Over the years, I have been on numerous radio stations talking about cancer. For example, the BBC *Africa Have Your Say* broadcasting to millions on prostate cancer and again on erectile matters. TV work has included *Black Britain*, *London Live*, Sky TV news, an Independent television (ITV) documentary. One highlight was an appearance on the Sky 1 programme *An Idiot Abroad* starring Karl Pilkington and Ricky Gervais. My role was to perform a digital rectal prostate examination on Karl Pilkington. Although the programme is a comedic vehicle, it was an effective way of communicating a serious message about the prostate gland. The YouTube videos have garnered over 1 million hits. I have been recognised in public places and even had 'selfies' taken. More recently the BBC has filmed me in Nigeria and in London for a piece highlighting research in the two countries on prostate cancer. When I can, I lecture and teach in Nigeria. I often give free urological consultations, despite being ostensibly on holiday!

In 2013, I was honoured with a Member of the Order of the British Empire for services to urology and the NHS. I received the medal at Buckingham Palace from Prince Charles. 'Never a dull moment', as they say, and on looking back, I would take the same trajectory. My advice would be to diversify your interests and pursue further study and qualifications. I believe that if you work hard and help and support others, people will ask you to contribute in many ways, whether in the voluntary sector or teaching or committee work. Contribute where you can and do not rest on your laurels!

LEADERSHIP

Sir Sabaratnam Arulkumaran

Peter F. Drucker argues that 'leadership without direction is useless. . . . As the pace of change in our world continues to accelerate, strong basic values become increasingly necessary to guide leadership behaviour'. I believe clinical leadership is about imparting more than knowledge or skills, it is also to build future leaders – whether in practice, education, training or research.

In both undergraduate and postgraduate medical education, consultation with trainees has revealed a desire to excel across a range of skills and capabilities. This desire reflects the changing role of doctors in medicine. Importantly for readers, development of non-clinical professional domains should not be viewed as a distraction to a clinical career; rather, aspiration to enhanced roles, be they in subspecialty practice, management and leadership, education or research, is likely to facilitate greater clinical engagement [1].

For today's medical students and trainees, the health landscape in which you practice is changing. The times of individual and isolated physicians have been replaced with teamwork, interprofessional learning, leadership and research innovation. The importance of leadership in research cannot be overstated; today, this is judged on the strength of the institution, the quality and quantity of publications and PhD theses and the impact of these outputs as measured by significance and reach. Bear these factors in mind as you seek out research opportunities of your own.

In time, you may be required to show leadership in medicine, let the '7 Cs' guide you: commitment, compassion, courteousness, competence, communication, confidence and continuity of care. My own career has enabled me to work in diverse parts of the world, from Sri Lanka to Singapore to the United Kingdom; I have had the honour of leading a range of departments and institutions, including the Royal College of Obstetrics and Gynaecologists (RCOG) and the British Medical Association. A few principles that have served me throughout are as follows:

1. Am I ready? Self-evaluate to see whether you are suitable to take on a specific leadership position by way of knowledge, experience and personality that is needed.

2. Am I compatible? I study the vision and mission statements of prospective organisations, meet key people at its different levels to understand how the organisation functions and consider whether and in what way I could contribute to or enhance its status.

3. Planning is power. It is essential that you formulate early plans on what steps are needed when you take the position.

For example, before I applied for the role of professor and head of the Department of Obstetrics and Gynaecology at St George's Hospital in London, I visited the institution four times and met with consultants, midwives, registrars, administrators, scientists and students. I formulated plans to improve teaching, research and clinical services. Once in post, to achieve maximal cooperation and productivity, I worked to enhance the self-esteem of consultants, encouraging and supporting them to run national postgraduate courses, conduct research or edit academic books, or join committees of the Royal College.

As president of the RCOG, I had a five-point plan:

- What can I do proactively, i.e. new things to improve women's health such as introduction of maternity dashboards.

- What can I do reactively, i.e. reading the recommendations of confidential inquiries of maternal deaths and producing new guidelines or improving those existing?

- What actions can be taken to develop leadership within the organisation and promote financial stability?

- How best to challenge members of the organisation to do better, e.g. introduction of good practice guidelines such as 'the responsibility of the consultants on call'?

- And finally, how to foster continuous engagement with the public, politicians and membership via different channels to maintain their support to improve women's health?

This short reflection offers some insight into how to approach leadership in medicine; and despite the scale of change that will occur in your lifetime, I hope you and, in time, your students will be reminded of Plato's timeless statement on the ideal leader – 'someone who commits himself to a life of service to fellow citizens'.

Reference

1. Tooke, J. *Aspiring to Excellence*. Medical Schools Council, London. 2008.

HUMANITARIANISM

Jim Ryan

So you want to be a humanitarian volunteer?

> Arrive, work and leave in a spirit of humility.
>
> **Anon**

Today, the delivery of humanitarian aid is as dangerous as ever. Confucius' phrase 'May you live in interesting times' now seems very apt. However, this should not deter you from considering a humanitarian mission. My own involvement began shortly after qualifying. I was a green regimental medical officer in the British Army with a parachute battalion on exercise in Northern Kenya when I was sent up country to assist a community beset by famine. I was woefully unprepared and could do very little. Here is my first piece of advice: never embark on an assistance mission if you are untrained and poorly equipped. The exhortation 'something must be done' must not guide your efforts. Box 10.1 lists some things you *must not do*.

Box 10.1   What not to do in humanitarian work

1. Wing it.
2. Go in on a wing and a prayer.
3. Have a go.
4. See one, do one, teach one.
5. Learn on the job.
6. Try something new!
7. Practice on the locals – they will not mind.

This early baptism of fire taught me a very hard lesson but one that would guide me in the future. The years that followed took me to Northern Ireland, Cyprus, the Falkland Islands, the Balkans, Middle East and the Caucuses. For these later missions, I was properly trained and equipped and had clear aims. These are absolute requirements if you are to achieve success and make a difference. My army career ended in 1994. I left with some regret but with the belief that the British Armed Forces now have a proven place in the field of humanitarian relief.

Having left the army, I embarked on an academic career. I was fortunate to be offered a chair at UCL, endowed by Leonard Cheshire International, part of the Leonard Cheshire Foundation, an international NGO with a presence in over 50 countries. The Leonard Cheshire International Trustees tasked me with establishing a department concerned with conflict and disaster medicine. This involved undertaking study missions to places as diverse as India, Nepal, Azerbaijan, Afghanistan, Sri Lanka, Bosnia, Kosovo and the Middle East. These missions also afforded me and my academic colleagues the opportunity to rub shoulders with a variety of non-government, government and international agencies in the deployed setting. Our main effort on these missions was not only to cast a cold, academic eye on the practice of humanitarian assistance in a variety of austere environments, but also to become involved in training and education. It was most revealing – most aid agencies worked with great humanity and skill and made a difference. But not all agencies achieved high standards. Another area of concern at this time was the gathering of a corpus of knowledge in the field and the establishment of humanitarian medicine as a legitimate medical discipline. This has now been achieved, as I will discuss.

As a medical student or in-training medic, there are now many avenues open for you to gain skills, experience and deployment in humanitarian medicine. Your earliest opportunity is to select a humanitarian module as a component of an intercalated BSc. At the time of writing, these are available in the United Kingdom at St George's, King's College London, UCL and the University of Birmingham. Oxford University will offer modules from 2017, and others will surely follow. After this, more formal accreditation can be achieved through diplomas and master's degrees. The Society of Apothecaries of London has a faculty of conflict and catastrophe medicine, established in 1994 and offers an internationally recognised diploma, with examinations taking place in the United Kingdom, the United States and the Netherlands. The London and Liverpool schools of tropical medicine and hygiene also offer highly reputable courses which may be required for humanitarian deployment. Alongside academia, other groups such as Medsin, Medact and the Royal Society of Medicine offer conferences and fora dedicated to humanitarian medicine. Finally, many reputable humanitarian agencies will offer internships to medical students which can provide an early entry point in the field, these include the WHO, the Office for Coordination of Humanitarian Affairs and the International Committee of the Red Cross.

It is important to consider the balance between your professional medical career and time spent with the humanitarian aid community. My advice is of a gradual involvement but always to see this work as very much a part-time commitment. Few people manage to work full-time in this field, and I would advise against it unless you choose a career in the Armed Forces. See Dr Jessica Tucker's excellent paper for further guidance [1].

In closing, do not expect to be deployed in your foundation and early training years. Most aid agencies will want you to be at least at specialist registrar grade or equivalent before they will accept you for an overseas aid mission. Quite apart from professional clinical competence, you will be expected to undergo rigorous personal preparation [2]. Physical and mental fitness are paramount. A history of cardiovascular, gastrointestinal or psychiatric illness will normally preclude deployment. Do not become a casualty yourself! Personal preparation should include home and family considerations. Consider matters such as wills and life insurance and settling your financial affairs. Do clarify with your insurance company that they will cover you in war and disaster environments.

Finally, consider also the effects of a long deployment on family life – tensions do arise. It is easy to forget that when you return home, you will need to pick up the threads of your personal and professional life.

I will finish by including a few pearls of wisdom gleaned from a generation of seasoned professionals in the field in Box 10.2:

Box 10.2   Wisdom for an aspiring humanitarian

1. Do your work in a spirit of humility and understanding – keep a low profile.
2. Take time to listen and understand the cultural mores of the people you are helping.
3. You are not a tourist. Be sensitive when using your camera – always seek permission.
4. Avoid displays of wealth and ostentation – do not offer gifts of money.
5. Do not make promises that cannot be kept.
6. Do not collect war souvenirs and keep away from unexploded ordnance (mines and other munitions).
7. Avoid illegal drugs and be temperate in your use of alcohol.
8. Be careful with your mode of dress.
9. Treat local staff with kindness and respect – listen when they offer advice.
10. Avoid political or religious comment and debate and keep away from political and religious rallies and meetings.
11. If provoked, be polite, patient and courteous.

Stay safe and bon voyage!

References

1. Tucker, J. Humanitarian work in the era of modernising medical careers. *Conflict and Catastrophe Medicine – A Practical Guide*, Ryan, J. M., Hopperus Buma, A. P. C. C., Beadling, C. W., Mozumder, A., Nott, D. M., Rich, N. M., Henny, W., MacGarty, D. (Eds.), 3rd Edition. Springer, London, pp. 929–38, 2014.

2. Millar, K. A. N. Accreditation in field medicine. *Conflict and Catastrophe Medicine – A Practical Guide*, Ryan, J. M., Hopperus Buma, A. P. C. C., Beadling, C. W., Mozumder, A., Nott, D. M., Rich, N. M., Henny, W., MacGarty, D. (Eds.), 3rd Edition. Springer, London, pp. 921–7, 2014.

CHAPTER 11

Afterword

Ashton Barnett-Vanes

In compiling this book, it has been a pleasure to interact with such a diverse and international cohort of medical students, junior and senior doctors and scientists. They offer a comprehensive series of chapters on making the most of medical school and training thereafter.

When addressing interns of the White House in 2016, the 44th president of the United States Barack Obama reportedly told them to 'worry less about what you want to be, and think more about what you want to do'. This is terrific career advice.

However, if you know what you want to do, how do you crack on with doing it? Proactivity is probably the single most underappreciated quality behind individual or collective success. In reading these pages, you will have gathered many insights and tips to interpret and apply towards your own ambitions. But – paraphrasing Newton's Third Law – nothing is going to happen until you act. So you decide to act, what next? Well, it might be plain sailing or it might bring you to the second half of Newton's Third Law: 'there is an equal and opposite reaction'. This could be from yourself, the *can't do* mentality or perhaps from other individuals and institutions resisting change.

Medicine is one of the most fluid and exciting fields to work in, a constellation of careers speaking a universal medical language focussed primarily on people's health and well-being. However, it understandably comes with an excess of historical baggage: many things done today have evolved from the precedent of days gone by as much as contemporary hard evidence. Accordingly, navigating and pushing this field forward can be challenging, and the temptation to keep your head down for five or six decades of your career is real. But what is life for if not to (gently) rock the boat now and again?

After all, where would modern medicine and surgery be without the genius of antibiotics? Or gender equity, without the invention of medical contraception? One day soon, cancer, HIV, dementia and a whole host of today's medical and social plights will be eradicated by the brilliance and determination of tomorrow's people – and you are one of them.

Index